Enhancing Compassion in End-of-Life Care Through Drama
The Silent Treatment

EWAN JEFFREY

and

DAVID JEFFREY

Foreword by
PROFESSOR STEVE FIELD
CBE FRCGP FFPH FRCP

Radcliffe Publishing
London • New York

Radcliffe Publishing Ltd
33–41 Dallington Street
London
EC1V 0BB
United Kingdom

www.radcliffehealth.com

British Library Cataloguing in Publication Data

A catalogue record for this book is available from the British Library.

ISBN-13: 978 184619 522 8

The paper used for the text pages of this book
is FSC® certified. FSC (The Forest Stewardship
Council®) is an international network to promote
responsible management of the world's forests.

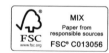

Typeset and designed by Darkriver Design, Auckland, New Zealand
Printed and bound by TJI Digital, Padstow, Cornwall, UK

Contents

Foreword

In times of moral complexity, uncertainty and fear, when is it appropriate to speak and when should one keep silent? *The Silent Treatment* explores clinical practice through a range of dramatic works and finds parallels between tensions in the plays and a modern end-of-life-care context. This is a timely moment to consider how a doctor may enhance their compassion as pressure is placed on the government to reconsider Physician-Assisted Suicide legislation and funding for the Arts is being reduced.

The book isolates dilemmas and crises that doctors, patients and their families may face, as reflected in the plays, and puts forward proposals for particular 'models' of compassionate care. For example, in Arthur Miller's *All My Sons* the writers observe a critical historical failure of a father to speak out against negligence and how this exerts pressure on his family in the present. Gurpreet Kaur Bhatti's *Behzti* explores the threat to a young Sikh woman's autonomy by a group of clerics who abuse their power and exploit the 'silence' in their closed community. Understanding these dynamics may help the medical team to develop their skills of empathy, compassion and communication.

Enhancing Compassion in End-of-Life Care Through Drama: The Silent Treatment is a valuable contribution to the field of end-of-life care, but also has a broad appeal to anyone interested in the symmetry between the challenges and opportunities of palliative care and the difficult moral and social problems that playwrights have explored over the ages, from the prescriptive power of State control in *Antigone* to the stark rendering of human resilience in the face of trauma in Sarah Kane's *Blasted*.

For many reasons it is often the case that doctors and the care team as a whole find it difficult to form a connection with a patient and their families, with their focus being primarily on practical arrangements and drug treatments, fearing that forming a bond with a dying patient may engender stress or even burnout. While this book takes the medical treatment plans into consideration, the writers admirably focus on what is less prominent in clinical training: how to develop one's compassion through a creative reading of theatre.

Ewan Jeffrey and David Jeffrey have written a compelling study of the intersections between dramatic narrative and the experience of the medical professional in end-of-life care. *The Silent Treatment* is a refreshing, accessible and human approach to what can be a daunting experience for the patient, the doctor and the medical team as a whole; and demonstrates how art can enrich and enhance, as well as providing an insight into the human condition.

Professor Steve Field CBE FRCGP FFPH FRCP

Deputy National Medical Director

Health Inequalities, NHS England

Chairman, National Inclusion Health Board

Immediate past Chairman, Royal College of General Practitioners

GP, Bellevue Medical Centre, Birmingham

May 2013

About the authors

Ewan Jeffrey

Ewan has worked as a Lecturer in Drama at Queen's Belfast since 2009. His teaching and research focuses on post-war British Theatre and Historiography, Drama and Medical Ethics and the plays of Harold Pinter, as well as writing for the stage and integrating audio narrative into contemporary performance and installation. Ewan's recent work has been staged across the UK and in Poland. Ewan wrote *The People Left Behind* featured in the Belfast Festival 2011 and based on a British Academy-funded multimedia research project on missing people and bereavement. He is interested in developing his integrated approach to sound and performance for future research projects.

David Jeffrey

David is an Honorary Senior Lecturer in Palliative Medicine at the University of Edinburgh. He was Academic Mentor in the Medical School at Dundee University until December 2012. He was a palliative care consultant in the Three Counties Cancer Centre Cheltenham after 20 years as a general practitioner in Evesham. He held a Winston Churchill Travelling Fellowship in 2006 and now is a member of the Advisory Council of the Winston Churchill Memorial Trust. David is a past Chair of the Ethics Committee of the Association of Palliative Medicine of Great Britain. His recent books include *Against Physician Assisted Suicide: a palliative care perspective* and *Patient-centred Ethics and Communication at the End of Life*.

'Surely human affairs would be far happier if the power in man to be silent were the same as that to speak.'

Spinoza, *Ethics*, Part III

'Whatever you have to say, say it in silence.'

Shashi Tharoor, *Riot*

Introduction

The British writer David Hare recounts an intriguing response that a friend had to one of his plays. Hare's *The Permanent Way* (2003) explores the disastrous effect of the privatisation of UK railways and the real-life accidents that stemmed from this mismanagement. He noted:

> The friend who came out of *The Permanent Way* – a play ostensibly about the privatization of the railways – crying because he saw it as being a play about AIDS in New York in the 80s had understood the play completely – because its true subject was avoidable and unavoidable suffering. This applies not just to railway crashes but all sorts of human stories. Great plays need metaphor: what method you use to achieve that metaphor is less important.[1]

This anecdote is pertinent to the issues we wish to explore in this book: namely how particular stories or narratives within a theatre context may enhance an understanding of suffering in a clinical context. There is nothing in *The Permanent Way* that is specifically about AIDS but for Hare's friend there was a subtext, a silent narrative that resonated deeply with him. We will in particular be investigating the use of silence within the plays, how it drives the plot forward and creates tension for the characters. In a similar vein we will explore how patients and healthcare professionals use silence in a clinical context. Doctors spend a great deal of time listening to patients' stories: one aspect of silent treatment. In palliative care these stories often relate to suffering, which doctors have a duty to do their utmost to relieve. To address suffering the doctor must be both competent, to deliver the best evidence-based treatments, and compassionate to engage with the individual patient's psychosocial and spiritual concerns. Compassion is therefore the vital element of the silent treatment and effective care. Concerns have been raised recently by nursing leaders, politicians and the media about a perceived lack of compassion in the delivery of care in the National Health Service (NHS). These concerns relate, not just to doctors and nurses, but also to management, governance and resources for patient care.[2,3,4,5] We are particularly concerned with exploring how healthcare professionals can improve their delivery of psychosocial and spiritual support to patients and their families. Although the clinical setting of this book is palliative care, and in particular end-of-life care, the learning points are relevant to all areas of clinical practice. Similarly, although some chapters focus on doctors the conclusions apply to all healthcare professionals. Our analysis is of topical interest as the chief nursing officer for England has recently launched a three-year strategy, 'Compassion in Practice', which applies to nurses, midwives and care staff.[6]

Good palliative care is concerned with relieving pain and other distressing symptoms and addressing the patient's psychological, social and spiritual concerns. Although the patient is the central focus of care, support of the family is an integral part of the palliative approach. Since the potential spectrum of a patient's distress can overwhelm the skills of any single healthcare professional, palliative care depends upon the involvement of a multidisciplinary team which may include: doctors, nurses, psychologists, spiritual advisers, social workers and other healthcare professionals. This holistic approach to the care of patients facing a life-threatening disease is relevant to all healthcare professionals, not just those working in specialised palliative care. As medical care has become more technical and the demand for treatment has increased, there is a risk that the psychosocial and spiritual elements of care become neglected. However, patients need healthcare professionals who are connected with them. Anatole Broyard says:

> I wouldn't demand a lot of my doctor's time; I just wish he would brood on my situation for perhaps five minutes, that he would give me his whole mind just once. I would like to think of him as going through my character, as he goes through my flesh, to get at my illness, for each man is ill in his own way.[7]

In Aristotle's *Poetics*, the philosopher places the two principles of *anagnoresis* (discovery) and *peripeteia* (reversal) and at the heart of drama. The diagnosis of an incurable disease represents both a discovery but also a series of reversals, losses, upheavals and crises. These crises will present physical, emotional, social and spiritual challenges for the patient, their family and their carers. *Enhancing Compassion in End-of-life Care Through Drama: The Silent Treatment* explores a broad range of plays from Greek tragedy to the present day and investigates how particular theatrical dynamics may help to understand complexities in the setting of end-of-life care. Just as Hare's friend found a poignancy and a uniquely personal context for *The Permanent Way*, we would like to explore different ways to interpret the action and subtext represented on the stage and find symmetries in a clinical context.

Drama is also concerned with exploring crises and change. There has been much research activity on the value of Applied Drama in a medical context, such as devising performance pieces to explore the experience of the patient, but comparatively little on the intersections between theatre *texts* and clinical practice. This interdisciplinary, collaborative work focuses on how 'canonical' theatre texts can inspire healthcare professionals to deliver improved end-of-life care.

In the range of plays we have chosen, the characters find themselves facing shock, uncertainty, upheaval and conflict. These critical situations are explored through a rich field of discursive expression: from the elaborate moral inquiry of Sophocles's *Antigone* to the brutal, intense honesty of English playwright Sarah Kane. Of course, the selection process of these plays was not easy, and the dramas themselves are challenging and often upsetting in their focus on suffering. Yet we wanted principally to explore key issues surrounding suffering and communication. The dialogue in these plays serves to map out key tensions in the human condition and the potential power of good communication to help and to heal in times of crisis.

The book will examine how silence and absence constitute both negative and positive elements in theatrical and clinical contexts; considering how a study of theatre might facilitate improved communication between patients, relatives and carers and how this might contribute to the education of healthcare professionals in the delivery of patient-centred end-of-life care. Sara Maitland, in *A Book of Silence*, comments that 'silence itself resists all attempts to talk about it, to try to theorise, explain or even describe it'.[8] She asks: 'is silence in the hearing or in the speaking?' We examine how this ambiguity is relevant to understanding patients and improving communication with them. We explore Maitland's hypothesis that silence is not simply a lack of language but something different from language; not just absence of sound but a presence of an entity which is not sound.[8]

This interprofessional analysis combines theatrical and clinical perspectives to create insights which can enhance compassion, and its component virtues: empathy, kindness and generosity. We hope that *The Silent Treatment* will contribute to improved patient-centred decision making in end-of-life care. The book aims to inform the education of medical, nursing and drama students and all healthcare professionals.

Each chapter of this book will focus on a play from a broad historical chronology. The different contexts and cultures in which the plays chosen for this analysis were written reflect a plurality which should be seen as strength rather than a weakness, since this mirrors the complexity of end-of-life care. Though we have given each chapter a key theme, such as Care or Connection, it is natural that there will be intersections between many themes both in the play under consideration and between the plays themselves. Compassion, for instance, is a theme which runs throughout the book and is explored in every chapter. It is hoped that we may pick up on some of these intersections as we explore the range of plays, in particular how the characters seek 'refuge' in the settings of the plays, only to find their environment is compromised by an uncaring outside world.

THE PLAYS

Good communication is at the heart of patient-centred care and is the cornerstone of a trusting relationship between the healthcare professional and the patient. The theme of communication pervades every chapter but the book begins by examining *King Lear* by William Shakespeare (1606). We investigate how elements of Shakespeare's *King Lear* might enrich our understanding of the challenges and opportunities of modern end-of-life care. One way of addressing suffering is to engage with patients and their families to find meaning in their new situation. For instance, Lear's decline into madness is followed by a degree of resolution as he discovers his humanity.

When disease is no longer curable the emphasis of treatment moves from cure to care, from prolonging life to improving the patient's quality of life. The focus of medical interest changes from the disease to the person. Notions of care are explored in *The Caretaker* by Harold Pinter (1960). Pinter's play explores interpersonal tensions which relate to family stresses during a terminal illness. This chapter interrogates notions of care, suffering, ownership and dignity. We also explore the consequences both of active intervention and a failure to act in two key sections of the play: when the character of Aston delivers a monologue concerning his own psychiatric institutionalisation (active intervention) and at the end of the play we observe a vulnerable old man, Davies, being rejected from his temporary home (failure to act). The fundamental areas of tension will be placed in a clinical context in terms of the dilemmas faced by the patient, family and healthcare professionals engaged in end-of-life care.

The relationship between the healthcare professional and the patient depends on a trusting connection between them. This 'connection' or mutual empathy is explored in *Journey's End* by RC Sherriff (1928). Sherriff's First World War drama is a compassionate and poignant study of a young recruit's deployment before a major offensive. Raleigh, initially full of patriotic optimism and in awe of Captain Stanhope, finds his illusions shattered by the brutal reality of life in the trenches. There are many intersections between clinical models of care and the action of the play (there is a particularly powerful scene where the characters remain crucially 'silent' over the killing of one of the officers). We also investigate how the soldiers find 'connections' between each other in terms of shared pasts and the distance between idealism and reality. Making sense of the past in order to confront or 'deal' with the future is a key element in both the plays and in the search for meaning in end-of-life care. *Journey's End* reflects the effects of chronic stress on the soldiers, a situation which is reflected in clinical care by doctors who suffer 'burnout'. This chapter explores ways in which doctors might look after themselves as well as their patients.

Patient choice has become a political mantra. The issue of choice is highlighted in end-of-life care in the current debate over the legalisation of assisted suicide and euthanasia. The debate is polarised between those who believe that patients should have the right to choose to seek help from doctors to end their lives and others opposed to this view who maintain that there must be limits to patient choice if that choice puts other vulnerable patients at risk.[9,10] *Antigone* by Sophocles (441 BC) remains a crucial text in understanding suffering and the debilitating power of social and religious mores that can disempower the individual and lead to ill-considered choices. In the play, pressure is placed on all of the characters (through both personal circumstances and a rigid, oppressive state ideology) to make choices without crucial insight or knowledge that might cause them to reconsider. In a clinical context the play can demonstrate how an ostensibly 'correct' choice can spark negative consequences and lead to regret and resentment in both patients and their families.

Successive NHS reorganisations have created challenges to ensuring continuity of patient care in the midst of recurrent changes. A study of *Little Eyolf* by Henrik Ibsen (1894) reveals the devastating impact of the loss of a child on a marital relationship. The play focuses on the death of Eyolf, the disabled son of Rita and Alfred. Eyolf drowns in the sea due, we infer, to the negligence of the couple. The play maps out the landscape of grief, blame and anger that accompanies bereavement and particular considerations in facing up to the death of a child. At the same time, *Little Eyolf* ultimately focuses on the possibility of renewal and accepting loss, thus exploring the idea of 'continuity' in the most distressing of changing circumstances. The chapter will focus on expectation and the human response to unanticipated change. Alfred's hopes for his son's future are dashed, just as the couple later find their marriage challenged by the burden of responsibility for the tragedy. Not only can *Little Eyolf* inform our understanding of the endurance of the human spirit, it can also highlight how we confront and adapt to loss and change.

Palliative care is care which is both competent and compassionate, and it depends upon honest information. Issues of professional silence or concealment of the truth are highlighted in *All My Sons* by Arthur Miller (1947). Miller skewers the American Dream in this uncompromising rendering of a small town family during the Second World War. The father, Joe Keller, has been exonerated over the sale of defective aeroplane machinery, the blame having fallen on his business partner. The play tracks the tensions that emerge within the family as the truth of Joe's dealings begins to emerge, causing the damaged but devoted father to commit suicide in the play's poignant denouement.

Miller challenges notions of 'collusion' with a particular focus on the pressures that are exerted on family members to conform to unrealistic expectations. Crucially, Joe has stayed silent about the truth of the business transactions because he feels it will compromise his identity both as a father and as a career man. The play has parallels with examples of collusion, both from the medical team and from patients and their families, in making key decisions about their care.

Care involves cooperation between the one who is dying and the many who care. *Blasted* by Sarah Kane (1995) is an audacious and controversial play, written in the wake of the 1995 Srebrenica massacre. It interrogates bourgeois complacency and the human tendency to distance oneself from the suffering of others. Ian, a racist foul-mouthed journalist, and his exploited 'girlfriend' Cate are staying in a luxury Leeds hotel when the building is hit by a bomb and the couple find themselves in the middle of a vicious and bloody civil war. The arrival of a brutal, battle-scarred soldier creates a situation of mutual dependency where the characters struggle for survival. The play is graphic in its depiction of violence and sexuality, but it is also ultimately humane.

There are many parallels here that can be drawn with how we view (or choose not to view) 'suffering' in the context of terminal illness. Like Kafka's novella *Metamorphosis*, Kane is interested in the temptations to maintain a form of 'silence' over the plight of others. When Ian and Cate find themselves confronted directly by a situation that has previously been peripheral to their experience (such as manifested in news headlines), they find that they can no longer remain silent but must engage and attempt to understand the harrowing circumstances for themselves. In a clinical context we explore the psychosocial and spiritual aspects of the crisis of dying. The play gives insights into the emotional responses which may surface in an existential crisis. Ian's personality appears to change from swaggering bully to someone who is vulnerable and compromised. The play ends with a note of optimism, with Cate looking after the grievously wounded Ian who both communicates warmth to Cate and finds an understanding of his situation. We investigate the notion of 'a good death' in the clinical setting and suggest ways of helping patients facing such existential crises.

Cloud 9 by Caryl Churchill (1979) is a subversive drama which explores issues of complexity, colonialism and the social construction of one's identity in terms of race and gender. The play follows the same family in two (apparently) radically different contexts. The first is 19th-century colonial Africa, the second is late seventies Britain. All of Churchill's characters harbour secrets concerning their 'real' identity. Churchill partially achieves this by specifying, for example, that some male characters should be played by females, children by adults and the black character by a white actor.

Churchill's play is both critical of the way in which prejudices are constructed and how individuals are disempowered by social 'categorising'. The play can help us understand how patients defy expectation and need to be treated as individuals rather than products of a particular social context. *Cloud 9* both reinforces the need for confidentiality while at the same time exploring the need for transparency in human interaction. Palliative medicine is not highly technological care but it is highly complex care. It challenges healthcare professionals with difficult ethical dilemmas and complex psychosocial communication problems. We explore notions of complexity in *Cloud 9* and relate our ideas to end-of-life care.

Cultural influences in caring for dying patients are addressed in an analysis of *Behzti (Dishonour)* by Gurpreet Kaur Bhatti (2004). *Behzti* is a play that explores cultures of silence. Min, a young Sikh woman, must care for her sick mother Balbir while dreaming of escaping her repressive existence with her young lover Elvis. Torn between filial and religious duty, she finds herself in a still more vulnerable position when she is pressurised by the sinister senior cleric Mr Sandhu. What is important here is that the analysis is not specifically focused on the pressures of organised religion but more on the tensions between public and private life and expectations of 'responsibility' in caring for sick or dying people. It is sad that some ethnic minority groups do not access specialist palliative care services to any great extent. We look at possible reasons for this inequality in healthcare provision. A study of *Behzti* can also inform clinicians' responses when helping people from differing cultural backgrounds grapple with their impending death.

Patient-centred care may be threatened by well-meaning medical paternalism. One powerful mechanism of limiting paternalism and enhancing patient autonomy is a requirement for the patient's informed and understood consent to any medical intervention. So why *The Silent Treatment*? A particular focus will be placed on the role of silence within both the plays and in the clinical context. In many ways, silence can be seen to be damaging in human interaction. Pinter's famous pauses, for example, create an atmosphere of unease, moments of vulnerability when words cannot be used to screen the characters' insecurity. But for doctors, there are times when it is necessary to stay silent. We can observe how crucial silences in the past have damaged Joe Keller's family in *All My Sons* and find similar dynamics in end-of-life care. Communication, clarity and honesty are vital in a clinical context. Yet we would like to propose, in the final chapter of the book, that some of the most important aspects of end-of-life care are realised through silence: through non-verbal communication. Compassion cannot be generated simply by 'saying the right things'. Some of the most powerful moments in the plays which we examine are those that take place without dialogue, from Cate's compassionate feeding of the wounded Ian in *Blasted*, to Stanhope's comforting of the dying Raleigh by simply moving a candle nearer his bed in *Journey's End*.

We recognise that these plays have been written in different historical periods and from writers with different cultural and social backgrounds, but propose that we may find useful links not only between the narratives but synergies with the challenges (moral, social and ethical) that doctors will face in end-of-life care. Please note that this book is not meant to be prescriptive or exhaustive but rather act as a springboard for a wider consideration of how theatre can help doctors understand the dynamics and demands of end-of-life care. We would urge readers, if possible, to attend performances of the plays: after all, a theatre text is only a formula for an act that should be live and engaging in the spirit of the moment.

We hope that this book may be of value in a range of educational contexts. There is broad agreement that medicine has much to learn from a study of the arts and humanities but little consensus as to the best way to bring this about. Healthcare professionals spend much of their time listening to stories of sickness related by patients and their families. It thus seems appropriate that drama, which is primarily concerned with exploring narratives, change and crises and relies, like the clinical situation, on communication, is an ideal medium for healthcare professionals to gain new insights into care. A chapter looks at teaching methods in a drama workshop for medical students. We aim to examine problems and opportunities that the plays can present in a workshop context and each chapter ends with a model which summarises some of the main concepts discussed.

Our final chapter combines the insights and questions raised by the previous chapters to reflect on how these impact on medical professionalism. We try to answer the question: What is a good doctor? We would like to think that this book will be relevant to all healthcare professionals who work with patients, not simply those involved in hospices and other areas of specialist palliative care. The word doctor is derived from the Latin *docere*, 'to teach' and in acknowledging the core role of teaching we have addressed the ways in which these plays might be used as a valuable educational resource to clinical teachers, particularly as an inspiring way to enhance professional development.

Overall, we hope to show how theatre texts engender creative problem-solving ideas which promote an empathic approach to end-of-life care. Like the plays themselves, the book will present questions rather than answers which, we hope, will provoke reflection on the complexities of end-of-life care.

REFERENCES

1 Hare D. David Hare live webchat – post your questions here. *The Guardian*. Available online at: www.guardian.co.uk/culture/theatreblog/2012/mar/21/david-hare-live-webchat-questions (accessed 17 January 2013).

2 Siddique H. Nurses told to focus on compassionate care. *The Guardian*. 4 December 2012. Available online at: www.guardian.co.uk/society/2012/dec/04/nurses-compassionate-care (accessed 14 December 2012).

3 Hill A. Winterbourne View Care Home Staff jailed for abusing residents. *The Guardian*. 26 October 2012. Available online at: www.guardian.co.uk/society/2012/oct/26/winterbourne-view-care-staff-jailed (accessed 14 December 2012).

4 Curtis P, Mulholland H. Panorama care home abuse investigation prompts government review. *The Guardian*. 1 June 2011. Available online at: www.guardian.co.uk/politics/2011/jun/01/panorama-care-home-abuse-investigation-government-review (accessed 14 December 2012).

5 Campbell D. Neglect and indignity: Stafford hospital inquiry damns NHS failings. *The Guardian*. 1 December 2011. Available online at: www.guardian.co.uk/society/2011/dec/01/stafford-hospital-inquiry-nhs-failings (accessed 14 December 2012).

6 Department of Health. NHS Commissioning Board. *Compassion in Practice*. December 2012, London: DoH. Available online at: www.commissioningboard.nhs.uk/files/2012/12/compassion-in-practice.pdf (accessed 14 December 2012).

7 Broyard A. Doctor talk to me. *New York Times*. Available online at: www.nytimes.com/1990/08/26/magazine/doctor-talk-to-mehtml (accessed 17 November 2012).

8 Maitland S. *A Book of Silence*. London: Granta; 2008.

9 Jeffrey D. *Against Physician Assisted Suicide: a palliative care perspective*. Oxford: Radcliffe Publishing; 2008.

10 Warnock M, Macdonald E. *Easeful Death: is there a case for assisted dying?* Oxford: Oxford University Press; 2009.

CHAPTER 1

Communication: *King Lear*, William Shakespeare (1606)

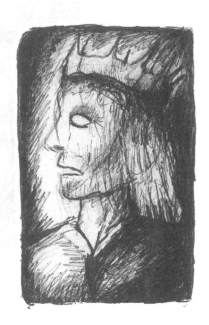

'Unaccommodated man is no more but such a poor, bare, forked animal.'

King Lear

INTRODUCTION

King Lear was first performed at the court of King James I on 26 December 1606. 'It was played before the Kinges Maiestie at Whitehall vppon St. Stephans night in Christmas Holidayes.'[1] The original story of King Lear would have been familiar to many in the first audience. Yet Shakespeare's play departs from the original myth and represents the darkest and most cruel of all his tragedies, but one which continues to have an enduring hold on our imagination in its depiction of resilient humanity in the face of despair.

King Lear's contemporary resonance spurred the playwright Edward Bond to adapt Shakespeare's play in order to draw parallels with how we respond to, or turn away from, violence and destruction today.[2] Shakespeare's original narrative, however, in its exploration of grief, loss and suffering, also provides startling insights which can specifically inform modern end-of-life care.

In this chapter we would like to examine primarily the issue of communication as the cornerstone of good practice and to identify the extent to which the characters communicate or fail to do so and to draw parallels with the clinical context. Central to the issue of communication is the negotiation of silence, of knowing when to speak, and when to remain silent, and this holds true for *King Lear* and the other plays we will examine in later chapters. *King Lear* is a play that derives much of its theatrical tension from miscommunication, from the initial, tragic failure of the king to understand Cordelia's remarks in the opening stages, to the later conversations between the king and the blind Gloucester.

In a later chapter we will examine how a person's ontological security (the belief that life will carry on as normal, and that they are impervious to major change) can be challenged: Chapter 7 focuses on Sarah Kane's *Blasted* in which a couple whose 'comfortable' existence in a hotel is literally blown apart by a bomb. Likewise, Lear believes himself to be infallible and all-powerful, yet he finds himself experiencing life-changing suffering. In a medical context, a diagnosis can place a patient in a position of despair and fear; it is the aim of the palliative care team to assist in managing this fear and to conserve the patient's dignity.

PLAY SYNOPSIS

The ageing King Lear decides to divide his kingdom between his three daughters. His youngest daughter Cordelia is disinherited and the kingdom is divided between her sisters Regan and Goneril. Kent defends Cordelia and so is banished by Lear.

In a sub-plot Gloucester is deceived by his bastard son Edmund, forcing Edgar his legitimate son to leave and feign madness as a beggar.

Lear quarrels with Regan and Goneril and departs into a raging storm on the heath with his Fool and Kent disguised as a servant. Gloucester helps Lear but is betrayed by Edmund and is tortured by being blinded by Regan and her husband.

Lear is taken to Dover where Cordelia has landed with a French army, which is defeated. Edmund is forced into a duel with an unknown champion who fatally wounds him and reveals himself to be Edgar. A dying Edmund orders the death of Lear and Cordelia and then admits his crime. Furious attempts are made to prevent Cordelia's death, but too late, the order has been carried out. Lear, overwhelmed by grief, dies beside Cordelia.

CLINICAL CONTEXT

We investigate how elements of Shakespeare's play might enrich our understanding of the tensions, challenges and opportunities of end-of-life care. For while it is possible to dwell upon the bleaker aspects of *King Lear* and view the play as uncompromising and depressing, it is equally viable to see how the play celebrates the human spirit in the face of persistent adversity. Lear finds a sense of self-worth and, arguably, final resolution at the end of his life through, and not despite, challenging circumstances. Similarly, patients can often find reconciliation and meaning at the end of their lives and in so doing can also achieve a 'good death'.

The play opens with King Lear disinheriting his youngest daughter Cordelia because she will not publicly express her love for him as was expected by social conventions of the time. Cordelia expresses her true feelings rather than conforming to court protocol and enrages Lear when she tells him she cannot compare the love she has for him with anything; she is then banished from the kingdom. When we come to look at Harold Pinter's *The Caretaker* in Chapter 2 we will examine how again language can in fact be a barrier rather than a method of clear communication.

King Lear represents the king's development from an arrogant figurehead to a human: 'a very foolish fond old man' who finally gains self-awareness. Shakespeare's play confronts us with our own mortality and in doing so interrogates related notions of suffering, pain, family and identity: all concepts which are central to palliative care. In Edward Bond's adaptation of Shakespeare's play, a soldier tells a tortured and mutilated prisoner (a counterpart to the blind Gloucester) 'You'll live if you want to.'[2] Gloucester, after being blinded and discovering Edmund's treachery, remarks: 'I stumbled when I saw.' While neither Bond nor Shakespeare are glibly suggesting that traumatic events can have a positive impact, their representations of the Lear story show how suffering may bring with it a form of catharsis and understanding of our own and others' vulnerability and in doing so generates compassion.

Further, Shakespeare consistently uses inverted notions of vision and blindness as, respectively, metaphors for enlightenment and lack of clarity concerning the human condition. No character in Shakespeare's play is able, completely, to 'see' clearly and thus find complete reconciliation, but the playwright shows us how when physical damage is inflicted on the person there can also be a form of psychological healing and resolution.

At a primary level, Shakespeare explores communication in the context of family life and in particular the bond between father and child. 'The bond cracked 'twixt son and father.'

The play effectively begins with Lear planning his retirement:

'tis our fast intent
To shake all cares and business from our age,
Conferring them on younger strengths, while we
Unburdened crawl toward death

However, his bequest of a kingdom is conditional upon a public declaration of his daughters' love. Cordelia's refusal to take part in this charade causes her to be banished by Lear: 'Hence and avoid my sight!' The loyal Kent tries to make Lear recognise the potential treachery of Regan and Goneril's rehearsed answers: 'Kill thy physician and thy fee bestow upon the foul disease.' As so often occurs in clinical practice when breaking bad news, Kent suffers the rage vented against the bearer of the bad tidings and is also banished. The fear of rejection by the patient may be a factor preventing healthcare professionals (and family members) from the honest discussion that would help patients and families plan their future care. Similarly, patients may conceal emotions such as anger for fear that they may be rejected by the professionals on whom they depend.

Parents often quarrel with the children they most resemble. When the vain Lear gives away his kingdom he expects gratitude from his daughters. Regan and Goneril are both cruel and cunning, and when Lear realises the depths of their treachery, he is driven mad with anger and grief. 'Thou better knowst the offices of nature, bond of childhood, effects of courtesy, dues of gratitude.'

They have broken the bond between parent and child which is one of the fundamental moral tenets in society. When we are young our parents seem as omnipotent as was King Lear in his prime, but as we mature we become aware of their vulnerability. Regan and Goneril, in their actions, are monstrous, but they serve to illustrate the ambivalence which may lie beneath the surface of the child–parent bond.

When a parent is dying the family are under great stress and may feel guilt, anger and helplessness. In these circumstances it is hardly surprising that healthcare professionals can be faced with families quarrelling around their dying relative. The distressed family may vent their anger by making complaints about professional carers. Similarly, ageing parents may find it difficult to accept physical help from their children. Indeed, there is palpable tension in the play when Lear's 'Fool', or surrogate son, appears to have a world-view that is more balanced and mature than that of the king himself.

Shakespeare's stark description of dysfunctional family dynamics serves to warn healthcare professionals against the unrealistic hope that they will be able to resolve all conflict. He helps them to understand the reasons why families may behave in these ways.

But Lear's relationship with his biological relatives is only one dimension of the concept of family that may inform both an understanding of the play's dynamics and those at the heart of palliative care. Lear's rancorous relationship with his daughters is contrasted with his surrogate 'family' of Gloucester, Edgar, The Fool and Kent. Just as it may be challenging for a palliative care team to understand the tensions in the biological family of the patient, they must also understand that they may be a 'family' to the patient. The palliative care team as the 'professional family' can also be dysfunctional at times, adding to the distress of the patient. It may also be difficult for the patient and their family to question the inaccessible and powerful 'professional family'. Thus the process of end-of-life care is, as in *King Lear*, an interaction between two families: the biological and the professional.

CASE HISTORY: PROFESSIONAL AND BIOLOGICAL FAMILIES

Robert is a 45-year-old electrician married to Karen (42); they have two teenage children Douglas (17) and Moira (15). Robert was diagnosed with lung cancer six months ago, which unfortunately was inoperable. He wants to remain at home despite now being confined to bed.

Robert's GP is Dr Penny who is now visiting him at home once a week. The district nurse, Abigail, visits each day as do the home care assistants who come in for a couple of hours to give Robert his personal care. Karen has become exhausted looking after Robert and keeping up her job as a primary school teacher. Dr Penny suggests that Robert could be admitted to the local hospice to give Karen and the family a break. Karen disagrees with this idea and thinks it would be better if more support could be given to Robert especially at night but is frightened to contradict the GP.

While Abigail is visiting, Karen is able to raise these concerns about Dr Penny's management plan. They both go in and speak to Robert who says he would much prefer to remain at home to die. Abigail says that she will discuss their concerns with Dr Penny and suggests putting in more home care nursing in the evening and a Marie Curie nurse to stay overnight for few nights to give Karen a rest. Robert and Karen are much happier with this plan.

When Abigail informs Dr Penny of their concerns and her ideas for putting in extra support he is initially angry. 'Why didn't they say anything about this to me?' he asks.

Abigail explains that because the family knew her better from her frequent visits they were able to raise their concerns without fears of being seen as difficult. Once Dr Penny realised that what was important was that Robert and the family achieved the best outcome, he thanked Abigail for acting as an advocate for Robert and Karen and he arranged the extra support. This enabled Robert to remain at home until he died peacefully a week later.

SUFFERING

We would like to explore the notion of suffering as a failure of communication, as a feeling of being disconnected from oneself and others. Frank suggests that suffering involves experiencing life which is 'not as it should be' and there does not seem to be any way of restoring the past.[3] Suffering encompasses loss and the anticipation of loss, and is often hard to articulate and to define. While suffering is not limited to illness, life-threatening illness can be a time of suffering. Much of suffering is silent and this is one reason why doctors sometimes need to refrain from attempting to explain suffering yet not abandon the patient; a doctor's presence in itself can be a comfort. 'Watch with me' was Jesus' plea to his disciples in Gethsemane on the eve of his crucifixion. This was not an unrealistic demand to take away all suffering but an acknowledgement of the comfort derived from the presence of another human being at times of crisis. While we may view Lear as the central character in the play, it would be naive to claim that Lear alone suffers. Likewise, it is not uncommon for the relatives of a terminally ill person to be more distressed than the patient.

Furthermore, some of the most acute suffering experienced by the patient is caused by the anticipation of future incapacity. At the very end of Act 1, Lear makes the first reference to madness: 'O let me not be mad. Not mad, sweet heaven! I would not be mad. Keep me in temper, I would not be mad.'

This fear of mental deterioration is common among patients with advanced cancer and among the elderly. In Chapter 5 we will revisit this theme of the fear of madness in Ibsen's play about bereavement, *Little Eyolf*.

When, later, Lear is also rejected by his daughter Regan, he feels he has none of the dignity of old age. 'You see me here you gods, a poor old man, as full of grief as age, wretched in both.' It is evident that Lear feels he has brought shame upon himself, for mistaking Cordelia's honesty for treachery and thus bringing about his mental collapse. In Chapter 9 we will explore notions of 'honour' and 'dignity' within a particular community and investigate related cultural tensions that arise.

As the storm begins, Lear's preoccupation with his mental collapse is again evident: 'I have full cause of weeping, but this heart shall break into a hundred thousand flaws or e'er I'll weep. O fool, I shall go mad.'

While Lear dreads the onset of madness it is poignant that it is through this 'madness' that he gains insight into injustice, hypocrisy and his own humanity. He feels what poor naked wretches of his kingdom feel: hunger, cold and despair. 'The art of our necessities is strange and can make vile things precious.' King Lear has apparently lost everything: his daughters, his kingdom, his sanity. He even tears off his clothes. In terms of material wealth and the socially 'correct' relationship with his daughters he is bereft. However, in a sense he has gained everything, his insight into a shared humanity: 'Unaccommodated man is no more but such a poor, bare, forked animal.'

Suffering is a part of all illness and is an inevitable part of life. It is closely linked to loss either in the present or an anticipation of loss in the future.[3] Frank writes 'at the core of suffering is the sense that something is irreparably wrong with our lives, and wrong is the negation of what could have been right'.[3]

One of the challenges facing healthcare professionals is the fact that much of a patient's suffering is hard to articulate. As Frank has observed, some elements of suffering are negative and related to absence: what is no longer there, what is no longer right. This silent suffering can be addressed by doctors and nurses who are aware of their own emotions and appreciate the importance of presence, touch and silence in the therapeutic relationship.

Doctors engage with suffering as witnesses to the patients' stories. This enables the patient to share their experience of suffering. This role presents a challenge to the doctor to respond to the patient by developing a human relationship as well as a professional one.[4]

In this mutual relationship the doctor learns how hard it is to be a patient and the patient gains insight of the difficulties of being a doctor. Frank observes that some doctors do not acknowledge their need to be known as part of the clinical relationship. 'The pressure of being the one who is supposed to know is, of course, as enormous as it is isolating. By contrast, in knowing and being known each supports the other.'[4]

Patients facing a terminal illness also face a crisis which can involve many apparent losses. Like King Lear they feel that they have lost status and their plans for a comfortable future have been shattered. They may become isolated from family and friends. Shakespeare understood that suffering is not confined to physical pain but involves a loss of a sense of self and a loss of relationship with others. Such feelings of despair, helplessness and hopelessness can make some patients feel that life is no longer worth living. However, clinical experience suggests that the final stages of a patient's life may be a time of heightened self-awareness and an opportunity to find meaning and resolution.

Palliative care also involves engagement with suffering and a commitment to the individual patient that they will not be abandoned. This therapeutic relationship, which may take some time to develop, is a powerful way of understanding and relieving suffering. Edgar reflects that to be on one's own and suffering is much harder to bear than when the experience can be shared with others.

> Who alone suffers, suffers most i' the mind,
> Leaving free things and happy shows behind;
> But then the mind much sufferance doth o'erskip
> When grief hath mates, and bearing fellowship.

Doctors and nurses can help to relieve suffering by staying with the patient and continuing to affirm their value when there are no further active therapies available.

There are positive messages in the help that King Lear receives from Gloucester, Kent and finally Cordelia. Cordelia, his faithful daughter is reunited with the king. Briefly she has a feminine healing role:

> O my dear father! Restoration hang
> Thy medicine on my lips; and let this kiss
> Repair those violent harms that my two sisters
> Have in thy reverence made.

The brutal hanging of Cordelia in Act 5 leaves King Lear bearing her corpse onto the stage:

> Why should a dog, a horse, a rat have life,
> And thou no breath at all? Thou'lt come no more;
> Never, never, never, never, never.

In his terminal grief Lear expresses outrage that while his beloved daughter is dead even animals continue to live. But at the same time, the very fact that Lear can acknowledge that life goes on indicates that he has abandoned his self-centred view of the universe. His focus is now upon Cordelia; he finds her death unbearable and dies half believing that her lips moved at the moment of his death.

ASSISTED SUICIDE AND EUTHANASIA

Lear expresses terror at the thought of impending madness and suffering, yet finds healing and renewal as the play progresses. However, for some patients the prospect of future pain proves so overwhelming that they request assistance from their doctors to commit suicide. *King Lear* has valuable reflections on this difficult and sensitive issue.

Gloucester is blinded as punishment for helping King Lear. Wounded, he plans to throw himself off the cliffs of Dover. He is led by a beggar, Poor Tom, who is his loyal son Edgar in disguise. Gloucester is traumatised by both his blinding and by his discovery of his bastard son Edmund's deception. The disguised Edgar knows his father is full of despair but attempts to convince him to continue to live by tricking him into believing they have reached the edge of the cliff. He describes a huge drop in front of Gloucester, but there is in reality no cliff. Gloucester steps off, towards what he thinks is certain death, and falls to the ground at his feet. In his shocked state he believes he has landed on the beach a hundred feet below. Edgar in a different voice tells him he has survived a fall from the cliff top. Gloucester cries, 'Is wretchedness deprived that benefit to end itself by death?'

However, on further reflection he changes his mind, 'Henceforth I'll bear affliction till it do cry out itself, "Enough, enough", and die.' Later Gloucester again despairs and is urged to flee by his son. He replies: 'No further, sir; a man may rot even here.'

However, Edgar is not going to allow his father to give up, and responds: 'Men must endure their going hence even as their coming hither; Ripeness is all.'

This scene is possibly the hardest to explain. Why does Edgar keep up his disguise after he is reunited with his father? Although the deception surrounding Gloucester's suicide attempt is not the way in which doctors would respond to a patient's request 'Help me to die', the scene demonstrates that all lives have potential. In this case Gloucester comes later to learn that his son Edgar is alive.

Patients with a terminal disease may have suicidal thoughts but these frequently change with time and when they receive appropriate support. Individuals need to feel that they matter and that they are supported to have as good a quality of life as possible until they die.

At present in the UK there are those who are lobbying to legalise physician-assisted suicide. Some 400 years ago Shakespeare understood that we can never know what lies ahead and that even when life expectancy is limited, life is full of possibility. In Edgar's response 'Ripeness is all', the playwright draws an analogy between the suffering endured at birth and that which may occur in dying. Those working in palliative care share this sense of an appropriate time for death and are opposed to any move to legalise medicalised killing.[5]

Gloucester lives to meet King Lear in a powerful and moving scene. It is during this dialogue that Lear comes to appreciate his vulnerability: 'they told me I was everything; 'tis a lie, I am not ague-proof'.

APPROPRIATE TREATMENT

Shakespeare considers a complex ethical issue and one which raises difficult communication issues: the question of appropriate intervention at the end of life. When King Lear dies, Edgar steps forward to revive him: 'Look up, my lord.'

However, Kent stops him:

> Vex not his ghost; O, let him pass. He hates him
> That would upon the rack of this tough world
> Stretch him out longer.

Medical decisions at the end of life regarding withholding or withdrawing treatments are concerned with the difficult issues of balancing a wish to prolong life at any cost with a humanity which recognises that terminal diseases have a lethal power and it is sometimes appropriate to allow natural death. Medical technology has the power to prolong the process of dying; Shakespeare was aware that sometimes it is wiser to allow the natural course of events than always to intervene at the end of life.

These lessons are germane to palliative chemotherapy. Doctors need to consider whether it is ethically justifiable to use powerful drugs which may have considerable side-effects as a way of maintaining hope or because of a pressure to be seen to be doing something.[6] The greater use of palliative chemotherapy at the end of life may also be explained by patients and doctors mutually reinforcing each other's attitudes of 'not giving up'.[7] Nurses, on the other hand, tend to prefer allowing patients to make the best use of time left. This difference of view within the professional family can sometimes engender team conflict. In a Dutch study discussing death and dying with patients while at the same time administering chemotherapy was considered contradictory as this could diminish the patients' hope.[7] Inappropriate optimism about medical treatment plans at the end of life risks removing the chance for patients to confront their death and to prepare themselves and their family. Nurses, being closer to patients, often hear a different story from the patient, as the following case example illustrates.

CASE HISTORY: THE DIFFICULTY OF STOPPING PALLIATIVE CHEMOTHERAPY

Mary was a 60-year-old lady with advanced breast cancer. She had already received two courses of chemotherapy, but her disease was progressing with spread to her liver, bones and lungs. She had many side-effects from her last course of chemotherapy including hair loss, vomiting and fatigue. She met a specialist palliative care nurse at home and said that she had thought about things and had now decided that 'enough was enough'. She was going to ask the oncologist to stop her chemotherapy and spend more time with her family at home instead of visiting the hospital.

Mary went for her outpatient appointment and when the palliative care nurse rang her the next day to find out how things went, Mary replied, 'Oh, when I got there I had the blood test, everyone was so busy, it was easier just to have the chemo. I did not want to make a fuss.'

In a study of American oncologists, Jackson *et al.* showed that oncologists who viewed end-of-life care as an important role described communicating with dying patients as a process and reported increased job satisfaction. In contrast others who described their role in purely biomedical terms reported a more distant relationship with the patient, a sense of failure at not being able to alter the course of disease and an absence of collegial support.[8]

Breaking bad news is a process which may involve many conversations with the patient and their family. Acquiring the necessary communication skills to do this is not simply a matter of 'see one, do one, teach one' but involves a lifetime of practice and experience. Role models can help in this process and skills may be refined by using reflective practice. In this way the doctor gains in *phronesis* or practical wisdom and can see that she is a therapeutic agent. This willingness to listen and to talk about death and dying can be contrasted with society's denial and reluctance to engage with these topics. The sad consequence of making death a taboo subject is that it becomes to be viewed as a medical failure not as a natural part of life.

GENEROSITY: AN APPROPRIATE RESPONSE TO SUFFERING

Frank challenges doctors to increase the generosity with which they offer their medical skills.[9] He suggests that generosity comprises a welcome, consolation and an urge to meet the patient's needs. This spirit of hospitality encourages the ill to feel less stigmatised and isolated. A relationship of host and guest rather than provider and customer gives both parties the opportunity to take time to explore their real concerns. At the moment when two human beings share feelings of uncertainty, lack of resources and loneliness then a true dialogue is possible. As Dostoevsky wrote, 'Drop your tone and speak like a human being.'

Sadly, one encounters doctors who spend their time distancing themselves from suffering patients and adopting a dispassionate biomedical model of medicine, which treats the patient as a machine in need of repair. This behaviour demoralises both the patient and the doctor.

Suffering patients can be consoled by offering ways of actively planning the future, albeit a short one, and so giving this time a purpose. Viktor Frankl spoke of spiritual freedom which cannot be taken away and which makes life meaningful.[10] This freedom from attachment to things that are not really important, such as fame, possessions and ultimately our bodies, leaves us able to accept our situation and to live as fully as possible in the present. In meaningful dialogue between a doctor and patient each voice counts as much as the other and each is asking, 'What is it like for them from their perspective?'[9]

Generosity involves how we represent ill and disabled people and seeks their participation in decision making, in a true dialogue. Dying patients want a human relationship with their doctors and nurses; they don't want to be managed at a distance. If a doctor is to respond to a suffering patient in a humane way, they need to acknowledge that it is not possible to understand exactly how the patient feels and that we share vulnerability. The patient needs to be addressed, not talked about, and the doctor should talk like a human being, not using medical jargon or adopting a 'professional' distance.[9] Doctors who do engage with patients in a humane manner do not find this an extra burden but discover it makes work more fulfilling and much easier to bear.

A MODEL

These clinical concepts surrounding communication and suffering can be summarised by a model which links issues of suffering, connections, distancing and empathy.

A patient suffering a terminal illness may experience a number of emotions: despair, anger or helplessness. Doctors and other healthcare professionals have a choice when they meet such patients. They may respond to suffering in a positive manner by connection with the patient. Such engagement involves empathy, giving time and offering a listening presence. This connection helps to remind the patient that they still matter and their dignity is of concern to the caring team.

A negative way of responding to suffering involves the use of distancing tactics such as appearing busy, leaving the patient or restricting conversation to technical matters about the illness and treatment plan. This sort of behaviour makes the patient feel more isolated and increases suffering. The factors involved are summarised in the diagram below.

CONCLUSIONS

Nutall quotes a 'law': 'Whatever you think of, Shakespeare will have thought of first.'[11] *King Lear*, arguably the greatest tragedy ever written, has a power to provoke and disturb audiences today. Healthcare professionals working with dying patients and their families need to engage with their suffering and to

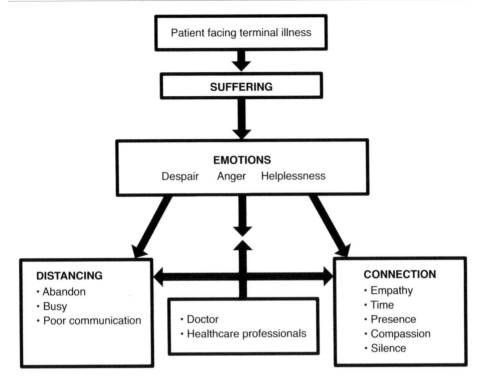

FIGURE 1.1 Model: responses to suffering

develop healthy ways of dealing with this stress. The most effective mechanism for this is through good team-working between the biological and the professional families.[15]

In *King Lear* we are not dealing with a single ethical dilemma but a play about the suffering of mankind.[12] Shakespeare describes the many dimensions of suffering: physical, social, psychological and spiritual. This concept was adapted by Dame Cicely Saunders in her writings on 'Total Pain'.[13] But can anything be learned from suffering? Edgar, Gloucester and Lear help each other and so become more humane in reassessing themselves and the society in which they live.

The fact that at the end of the play the three survivors, Kent, Albany and Edgar, are unwilling to take up the crown may suggest a negative ending. However, the men are abandoning an oppressive patriarchal system that champions convention and conformity over the individual's feelings. Edgar does not even attempt to articulate his grief but says that at this sad time they must say what they feel:

> The weight of this sad time we must obey;
> Speak what we feel, not what we ought to say.
> The oldest hath borne most; we that are young
> Shall never see so much nor live so long.

His last lines act as a warning that we should attend to and protect the emotional aspects of care.

In subsequent chapters, we would like to revisit particular themes that we have identified in *King Lear* and examine them in the light of end-of-life care. Of specific interest are the notions of social 'acceptability' (that Cordelia apparently defies), the transition from arrogance to awareness and the role of compassion.

Shakespeare's genius lies in his exploration of the ethical issues which underpin all human relationships without being overt in his position. King Lear resonates over four centuries for each new generation to gain insights into contemporary ethical and social challenges. Shakespeare explores 'the other', in spite of the difficulty that all social relationships are limited by the inaccessibility of others' minds. How do we know what other people are thinking, feeling and intending?[14] The answer is that much of our communication becomes a matter of interpretation and so there is always the possibility of error. In *King Lear*, Shakespeare takes a view that the 'self' is interactive and theatrical.[14] Interactive, in that a character's personality is a function of the other people they are interacting with, rather than a fixed nature. Theatrical, describing the differing roles the same person plays. Shakespeare's genius lies in observing and recording human behaviour. Shakespeare reminds us that we are always just an inch away from being 'a poor, bare, forked animal'. For Shakespeare the essence of humanity is fragility and thus our dependence upon others. Lear's journey from confident ignorance as king to hard-won insight is described as a tragedy. The tragedy lies in the loss and cost in gaining this insight. Lear is placed in situations of dependence on others which are totally unfamiliar to him. Tragedy begins when the character is inadequate to the situation he finds himself in; he is standing in 'boots that are too big for him'. Lear is deluded by the characters around him and loses his intellectual bearings.[14,15] The outward trappings of status and wealth are stripped away and a richer substance emerges: compassion.

REFERENCES

1 Ackroyd P. *Shakespeare: the biography.* New York: Nan A Talese; 2005.

2 Bond E. *Lear.* London: Royal Court Theatre; 1971.

3 Frank AW. Can we research suffering? *Qual Health Res.* 2001; **11**: 353–62.

4 Frank AW. Just listening: narrative and deep illness. *Fam Syst Health.* 1998; **16**: 197–212.

5 Jeffrey D. *Against Physician-assisted Suicide: a palliative care perspective.* Oxford: Radcliffe Publishing; 2008.

6 Munday DF, Maher EJ, Informed consent and palliative chemotherapy. *BMJ.* 2008; **337**: 471–2.

7 Buiting HM, Rurup ML, Wijsbek *et al.* Understanding provision of chemotherapy to patients with end stage cancer: qualitative interview study. *BMJ.* 2011; **342**: d 1933.

8 Jackson VA, Mack J, Matsuyama R *et al.* A qualitative study of oncologists' approaches to end-of-life care. *J Palliat Med.* 2008; **11**: 893–906.

9 Frank AW. *The Renewal of Generosity.* Chicago: University of Chicago Press; 2004.

10 Frankl VE. *Man's Search for Meaning.* London: Rider; 2004.

11 Nuttall AD. *Shakespeare the Thinker.* New Haven & London: Yale University Press; 2007.

12 Kermode F. *Shakespeare's Language.* London: Allen Lane Penguin Press; 2000.

13 Saunders C. The care of the dying patient and his family. *Contact.* 1972; **38**: 12–18.

14 McGinn C. *Shakespeare's Philosophy.* New York: Harper Collins; 2006.

15 Jeffrey E, Jeffrey D. Vex not his ghost: *King Lear* and end of life care. *J R Coll Physicians Edinb.* 2009; **39**: 15–19.

CHAPTER 2

Care: *The Caretaker,* Harold Pinter (1960)[1]

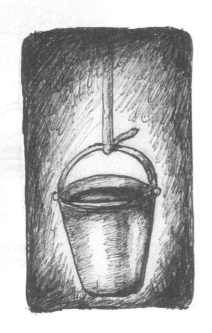

1   This chapter was first published as Jeffrey E, Jeffrey D. I could never quite get it together: lessons for end of life care in Harold Pinter's *The Caretaker. Journal of Medical Humanities.* 2012; **33**: 117–26. © Springer. With kind permission from Springer Science+Business Media B.V.

INTRODUCTION

> If Pinter's drama has not significantly influenced the modern dramatic
> form, it has had a profound effect beyond the theatre itself [...] Pinter's
> portrayal of human behaviour has affected how we view the behaviour of
> our fellow humans, who now appear not only to speak like his characters
> but also interact like them.[1]

Peacock's claim on the pervasive impact of Pinter's work on how we interact is
arguable, but his comment on the playwright's ability to make us view human
behaviour differently is astute. The stakes in Pinter's plays are always high, with
the characters struggling to keep a hold of a sense of personal identity while
mired in the quicksand of unreliable memories and the potential 'threat' of the
actions of others or unforeseen events. The tensions in Pinter's stagecraft may
be seen to have particular resonance in end-of-life care. In Chapter 10 we will
explore how we used this play in a practical context in a new module designed
to help medical students understand the challenges of end-of-life care through
drama and performance.

Harold Pinter's breakthrough play *The Caretaker* (1960) asks us to consider
the position of the individual who finds himself isolated, without connection, without being able – as one character puts it – to 'get it together' in the
face of the unknown (death or expulsion into the wilderness). This chapter
explores the symmetries between the characters' vulnerability in Pinter's play
and the position of the dying patient, their family and medical team in clinical care. Educational questions from both clinical and theatrical perspectives
are highlighted.

When exploring Pinter's work, it is important to recognise the central element of ambiguity (and sometimes opacity) that is a key dynamic in driving
the action of the play. But this should not be seen as a deficiency. We may be
used to listening to narratives which have a clearly defined beginning, middle
and an end; we may also expect to have any 'loose ends' tied up by the end of
the story. Yet this is hardly a reflection of the reality of our lives and while we
might identify with particular characters we might concede that certain plays,
films and novels offer us a form of escapism in their 'neatness' of plotting and
characterisation. Pinter's work is disturbing because it refuses to offer a notion

of 'escape', either for his characters who seem trapped in a frightening limbo; or for us as his audience, who have no easy cathartic ending or explanation. The critic John Somers takes an even starker view:

> Pinter appears to portray a world where there is no exterior authority and no overriding morality. The only value system seems to come from the room in which the protagonists move and the values represented and held by those, often threatening, people who come into it. There may be no 'outside' to which the characters can refer for guidance and help.[2]

There may well be symmetry here with the experience of end-of-life care where the patient finds himself/herself in a medical environment (and inherent 'system') which is unfamiliar and may at times seem threatening.

SYNOPSIS

The play is a complex three-way power struggle between a frail elderly homeless man, Davies, and two brothers in their thirties, Aston and Mick. The play opens with Aston kindly offering Davies a bed, although the dilapidated house appears to belong to Mick. Aston is quiet and withdrawn, and spends much of the play fiddling with an electric plug and talking about his goal to build a shed in the garden. Davies shows signs of being racist, appears selfish and manipulative but these traits mask (or are indicative of) a profound vulnerability and fear for the future. Davies claims that his current precarious situation will all be resolved once he gets his 'papers' which are apparently being held in Sidcup. Mick, the final component of this edgy trio, is ostensibly smart, streetwise and loquacious but with an undercurrent of potential violence.

Like Samuel Beckett's *Waiting for Godot*, the narrative is driven by a protracted tension in waiting: the play develops the *characters* rather than the plot. Again, parallels may be identified here in the context of end-of-life care, which may be seen as a framework of interpersonal interactions with the patient and the medical team. Pinter's play demonstrates how, in a vulnerable situation, oblique or fractured interaction leads to the characters' disempowerment. The passing of time is signified by the ominous drip of water from the leaky roof that collects in a bucket that hangs over the stage.

Through the course of the play Davies struggles to keep his place in the house as he attempts to exploit possible weaknesses in the brothers' relationship. In the process we learn that Aston has suffered a brutal form of electro-convulsive treatment (ECT) against his will, but the key dramatic action of the play is driven by Davies' lack of self-awareness and his subjugation by Mick, who offers him the comfortable job of caretaker, a promise on which he later cruelly reneges. When Davies finds that Mick has been using him as the butt of a cruel prank in this way, he desperately tries to assert some power by taunting the traumatised Aston about the young man's ECT treatment and fragile mental state, and implying that he (Davies) has a stronger relationship with Mick. Consequently, having alienated himself from both brothers, Davies is finally asked to leave by Aston. The play closes with the old man pleading, in vain, to be allowed to stay.

MODERN INTERPRETATIONS AND CRITICAL CONTEXTS

Pinter asks us to consider the nature of 'care'. The play is a succession of transactions, of tacit agreements and threats. It is an elaborately constructed narrative that explores the tensions between notions of 'caring' and ownership – which includes the ownership of decisions. Davies and Aston both suffer when decisions are made which undermine their autonomy. The men have apparent 'goals' that will validate their identities (Aston building his shed, Davies getting to Sidcup for his 'papers', Mick renovating the house), but these are unrealistic aims. Because the characters spend so much time repeatedly asserting their intentions in order to find a sense of ontological security, they find themselves engaged in conflict with the other characters and this process becomes defensive and reductive. We sense Aston will never build his shed, Davies will not visit Sidcup nor will the house ever be refurbished. In Chapter 9 where we explore *Behzti* we will see how the character of Balbir, a disabled and bitter matriarch, places all her faith in a 'list' that a powerful Sikh cleric apparently has, a list which presumably comprises eligible bachelors for Balbir's daughter, Min. At the end of the play we discover that this 'list' does not exist; Balbir's fantasy, however, causes the acute suffering of her daughter.

Frank defines care as 'an occasion when people discover what each can be in relationship with the other'.[3] This definition highlights the need for a sharing of vulnerabilities and engagement in a dialogue. Palliative care aims to improve the patient's quality of life.

Calman proposes a model of quality of life based on the 'gap' between one's expectations and present experience.[4]

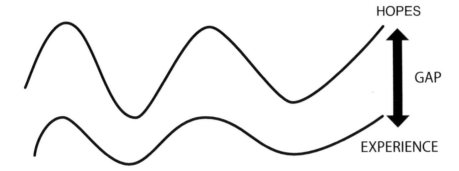

HOPES

GAP

EXPERIENCE

FIGURE 2.1 The quality of life gap (Calman[4])

According to his model, if, for example, a patient with advanced cancer is expecting to have as much energy as she enjoyed before she was ill, she will have a large gap between her expectations and her experience and will consequently feel she has a low quality of life. However, if she accepts that she will need to rest more and so reduces her expectations and conserves her energy for the activities she enjoys, the gap between her real experience and her expectation is small and she will feel she has a better quality of life. Calman's model has an important lesson for clinicians as it implies that as well as making the patient's experience, for instance pain control, as good as it can be, the doctor also needs to address the patient's expectations in a sensitive way and to plan realistic goals with them.[4] It must be remembered that the quality of life can only be described by the individual. It is unethical to make value judgements about the patient's quality of life. The doctor or nurse needs to have the skill to establish what the patient feels their quality of life is at any one time in the course of their illness. These assessments must be reviewed because patients change their views as their situation changes.[5]

Incidentally, Calman's model is interesting because it predicts the somewhat counterintuitive situation where a patient with cancer whose prognosis turns out to be much better than expected can feel unhappy and uncertain. In this case the reality is much better than expectations but the 'gap' between is wide.

Another key theme of *The Caretaker* – and one that imbues the play with much of its poignancy – is the unsettling way in which the distinctions between the individual, their territory and their property can be seen as arbitrary or can be manipulated by others. An example of this process is a scene in which Davies' bag is taken from him and passed back and forward by the two brothers while the old man frantically attempts to retrieve it. The bag becomes far more than just a personal 'belonging' and instead is representative of a person's autonomy, identity and power as an individual.

This 'blurring' of property and personal security can also be observed in a clinical context when a patient's autonomy is undermined by well-intentioned but paternalistic healthcare professionals. For instance, patients may have to wait for long periods before seeing a doctor, reinforcing a message that they are of less importance than the doctor who is always perceived to be 'busy'. Little account may be taken of the fact that time is of importance to the patient, especially in the context of end-of-life care. Patients often have their personal belongings removed when they are admitted to hospital and may have to talk to doctors when only partially dressed in a hospital gown. In these circumstances patients may feel undignified and their embarrassment and vulnerability effectively reduces their confidence to challenge any medical assumptions. In such a situation they are not equal partners in the decision-making process. The inequality of power between the doctor and patient may be symbolised by the doctor standing at the end of the patient's bed talking to a patient lying on their back. Doctors have enormous power and need to strive to share this power by ensuring that they communicate at the same level with a patient who is dressed and dignified. An open trusting relationship will be developed when the doctor seeks to see the world through the patient's eyes.

Active interventions can threaten a patient's autonomy and cause suffering, for example, during Aston's botched ECT treatment in the psychiatric hospital. But autonomy can also be threatened from a failure to act; for example, in the callous eviction of Davies where the character is left pleading to the brothers for his job and for shelter, but they fail to provide any care. These scenes resonate in the clinical setting of care, where patients may not be fully informed of the benefits and burdens of treatment or when they are discharged inappropriately from hospital.

Both Aston and Davies crave 'care' in a number of senses. They share a need for shelter, Davies is homeless and unemployed, and Aston who takes him in has a life goal to build his shed in the garden. These needs extend to seeking a haven from an uncaring world which threatens to strip them of their identity. It is this unknown that terrifies the protagonists and one which the stuttering Davies must face in the devastating closing scene. We all seek affirmation of our value and fear the unknown, emotions which are heightened at the end of life. This chapter will focus primarily on two key sections of the play where the notion of 'care' is abused: Aston's monologue and Davies' rejection.

Aston's monologue at the end of Act 2 offers an extraordinarily frank expression of the character's horrific treatment by the staff of a psychiatric hospital. The traumatic episode was triggered when Aston began to experience hallucinations, prompting him to say unsettling things to his fellow-workers and to diners in the nearby café.

The apparently vague opening to the monologue is carefully constructed so that the audience shares Aston's sense of disorientation. Many elderly patients experience a similar sense of disorientation in hospital, particularly when they are frequently transferred from one ward to another.

Aston's monologue is long, meandering and ambiguous in terms of detail. Is Aston unwilling (fearing a return to the hospital) or unable (through trauma) to explain precisely what he 'said' to these apparently avid listeners? What is certainly clear is that Aston's social framework found his symptoms and verbal responses objectionable and decided that he needed a form of enforced care.

We infer that Aston was sectioned, detained under the Mental Health Act, and subsequently received electro-convulsive treatment (ECT) against his will. The disturbing sense of flawed paternalism is intensified as Aston describes the hospital doctor giving him his diagnosis:

> 'You've got . . . this thing. That's your complaint. And we've decided, he said, that in your interests there's only one course we can take. He said . . . but I can't . . . exactly remember . . . how he put it . . . he said, we're going to do something to your brain. He said . . . if we don't, you'll be in here for the rest of your life, but if we do, you stand a chance.'

Aston's fragmented speech again displays both a sense of disempowerment and a persistent sense of ambiguity. He presents this meeting with the doctor as having an air of finality; there is no explanation in terms of the specifics of the illness or the treatment. As an audience, are we to apprehend that this was in fact a lucid and reasonable discussion that exists in a broken form in Aston's damaged memories, or is Aston faithfully capturing the opacity of this experience? In many ways, this is immaterial. What is crucial is that Aston's cumulative and pervasive experience is one where he has been deprived of his autonomy: it is not he who decides, but the shadowy medical 'we'. This supposed authority provides Aston with Hobson's choice. He can either have 'a chance' (although what this means is again left unclear) or he can live out his days in the institution. Aston comments that the doctor was a 'man of distinction', although he himself 'wasn't so sure about that'. Perhaps Aston trusted that the 'man of distinction' should have had his best interests at heart, but he was uncertain that this was the case. Patients may experience an ambiguity of feelings towards their doctors. On the one hand, patients may be grateful to doctors for care, yet they may, at the same time, resent the power of the doctor and their own sense of dependence on them. Trust between the doctor and patient is a cornerstone of good clinical practice, yet Aston reflects that no matter what good reputation the doctor may have, he does not trust him.

But if Aston is betrayed by the paternalism of the doctor, he also suffers at the hands of his mother who signs the approval form for Aston's barbaric shock treatment. Aston appeals to her for maternal care by writing to her – Pinter implicitly suggests she does not visit her son – but the doctor shows Aston the forms with his mother's signature, thus dragging any natural sense of familial protection into the arena of clinical bureaucracy. Aston then has no advocate to moderate the medical decision making; even his mother has rejected him. At best, the doctors have clearly failed to understand the relationship between Aston and his mother, at worst they have attempted to pressure her into providing her consent.

In a clinical context informed consent depends on a lack of coercion; the patient must be free to have time to reflect and to understand the issues before giving consent which is both informed and understood. In Aston's case he does not understand the potential benefits and harms of ECT. He is not allowed time or given an opportunity to question the doctor. If Aston is competent to give consent to the treatment, and there is no evidence of the doctor attempting to assess his capacity for decision making, another adult cannot legally give consent in his place.

Coercion is often present in more subtle ways in everyday practice. The busy nature of the ward round, the use of medical jargon, the presence of other patients waiting to be seen and the wish not to be a nuisance are all factors which can inhibit a patient from seeking full information or admitting that they do not fully understand what is about to happen to them. Informed consent is discussed in greater depth in Chapter 4.

The tension in Aston's monologue peaks in his account of the actual administration of the ECT. In defiance, he apparently climbed on the bed: apparently safe in the knowledge that the staff would not administer the ECT while he was standing. Yet the medical team went ahead with the procedure regardless. Again there is ambiguity that is generated both by the length of time that has elapsed since the incident, and Aston's damaged mental state: we cannot be certain if Aston's recollections are reliable and/or have become corrupted through his resentment at his forced incarceration and medical procedures that have not been explained to him. In a clinical context this again can manifest itself when trust is lacking, leading to a destructive sense of Them and Us in terms of the patient (and family) and the medical team.

After the 'treatment', Aston recalls he could no longer walk very well, and had trouble gathering his thoughts. He had reached the point where he 'laid out' his things in preparation for death. He claims at the close of his monologue, however, that he is now 'much better', but his introverted and distracted demeanour suggests otherwise. What is evident at every stage in this monologue is an insidious subversion of the notion of care from professionals who traditionally should act in a protective way but instead commit fundamental betrayals. This results in Aston being 'taken care of' while his narrative tracks his gradual disempowerment to a form of catatonia or living death.

It is crucial to note here that not only is Aston apparently betrayed by his friends, family and medical team, but in confiding in Davies about his past he unwittingly leaves himself vulnerable to a further betrayal by Davies himself, when the old man attempts to disclose Aston's traumatised state to disempower the younger man towards the end of the play. In many ways this is the most harrowing betrayal of all as we have assumed that Davies' silence during the monologue was at the very least due to some form of human sympathy. It is telling that this final betrayal is the one which prompts the normally docile Aston into demanding Davies' eviction. This scene emphasises the critical importance of confidentiality between the doctor and patient. The doctor is privileged to become aware of intimate details of the patient's story, particularly when patients are trying to discover a sense of meaning to their life. They would find it impossible to share this kind of sensitive information if they felt that it might be disclosed.

Aston's monologue provides insights into the plight of some patients with advanced cancer who opt for chemotherapy treatments which have only a very small chance of providing survival benefit.[6] Increasingly, chemotherapy is given closer to the end of a patient's life, so patients are making decisions about whether to accept such treatments while grappling with the knowledge of their impending death.[7] Even when they are informed that the goal of care is palliative, patients often feel that they have 'a chance' of prolonged survival if they opt for the treatment.[8] Patients need honest information to make rational decisions about their treatment. Some oncologists may fail to address issues of the survival benefits of palliative chemotherapy, preferring to talk in vague terms ('it may buy some time'), rather than confronting issues of death and dying with the patient.[9]

When cancer recurs and is no longer curable, active treatments may be withdrawn and so the patient may fear abandonment. This may be one motive for some patients to demand any sort of treatment for their cancer even if there is little evidence that it is beneficial. Patients may also feel that by continuing treatment they can focus on the management plan and then do not have to confront their dying.[9] In such situations palliative chemotherapy may be given to maintain hope.[7] In a recent national UK survey of deaths within 30 days of receiving chemotherapy, the advisory panel felt that in 19% of 649 patients the treatment was inappropriate.[10]

Doctors and nurses, like patients and their families, may find it difficult to stop active treatments and collude with patients to limit discussions to their treatment plan, thus avoiding confronting issues of death and dying.[9] A doctor may have feelings of failure or be overwhelmed by the pain of sharing feelings of loss when faced with a patient with unrelieved suffering. The doctor may feel that the only way to cope is to maintain what is sometimes called a 'professional' distance. At one extreme this could result in avoiding contact with the patient or at another level restricting conversation to issues of treatment plans. Learning to become aware of their own emotions in the clinical setting is an important task for doctors if they are to connect with patients and understand their concerns.[11]

Aston is taken to hospital without his consent. Ethical provision of care depends upon a requirement for informed consent, a process which acts as a mechanism for limiting the power of doctors to act in a paternalistic way, protecting the patient's autonomy. Although paternalism may be driven by good intentions to act in the patient's best interests, it does not take account of the patient's view and so threatens autonomy. Aston asks for further information about the proposed treatment but is denied, excluding him from decision making.

Aston admits his vulnerability in the key line: 'I could . . . never quite get it . . . together.' Patients in the terminal phase of their illness often have such feelings of vulnerability and hopelessness, feelings which can be addressed and relieved with good supportive care. There is a poignancy in Aston's feeble expressions of a desire for redress – of finding the man that 'did that' to him. Similarly, the relatives of patients who die sometimes complain about the patient's treatment; however, it may be that these complaints are an expression of their grief.

In Aston's treatment, at every level, the notion of 'care' is appropriated to 'treatment'. Instead of trying to empower Aston, his doctors take ownership of him and he is stripped of his independence. Aston does not understand why he is in the hospital in the first place, or the nature of his treatment. Effectively, the doctors maintain silence and do not communicate with him in any meaningful way. Further, Aston, having been abused in the hospital, no longer 'talks' in the café and has learned to live in a form of semi-silence. This failure of care by the doctors results in a stasis, a living death with no sense of closure. From a clinical perspective caring involves the capacity to connect with another person, to feel empathy for their situation; it is a physical, social and a moral activity.

Pinter's dramatic world in *The Caretaker* reflects many of the potential anxieties and tensions within end-of-life care. The characters are essentially in flux, the house is half-built and the weary Davies finds no space to rest. The three protagonists seek a form of connectedness or validation in a world that is shifting and uncertain: even the sinister Mick, after smashing Aston's Buddha in a rage, complains desperately of having 'plenty of other things to worry about'. Essentially, the characters find that they must 'take care' of difficult situations where in fact what they desire is to be taken care of themselves, but this 'care' does not materialise. It could be argued that Aston has been 'taken care of' in a sinister sense; active medical intervention has stripped him of his autonomy, his individuality and freedom.

DAVIES' REJECTION

When people become patients, they risk losing their autonomy and their dignity may also be compromised.[12] While active interventions in Aston's brutal treatment do not constitute care, a failure to act may also damage one's autonomy.

Tension arises within *The Caretaker* from the deceit of the characters and the setting of unrealistic goals. At the start of the play Aston offers Davies a place to stay 'till you . . . get yourself fixed up'. This collusion avoids discussing the reality that he will never get 'fixed up'. Patients' relatives sometimes ask doctors not to tell the patient the truth, in a collusion to pretend that things are not as serious as they really are. This collusion results in the creation of a barrier, so discussion about the fact that the patient is dying becomes a taboo. Doctors and patients themselves may collude by restricting discussion to treatment plans, so denying that death is inevitable. In society there is difficulty in discussing death and dying, some doctors have difficulty in accepting that death is a part of life, viewing death as a personal failure in their duty of care.

Aston then gives Davies a key to the house and to the room. Davies can hardly believe his good fortune, remarking, 'You're sure, you're sure you don't mind me staying here?' Having apparently found a place to stay, Davies is offered the job of caretaker, first by Aston and later by Mick. Davies starts to become confused, asking, 'Who's the landlord here . . . him or you?' Mick confirms that he is the landlord and Davies accepts: 'I don't mind doing a piece of caretaking.'

It is ironic that Davies is offered the post of caretaker when he is most in need of care himself. Indeed Aston and Mick need someone to care about them, but these needs are expressed only obliquely (the desire to 'fix up' the house or build the shed). In the clinical setting the needs of those taking care are commonly neglected whether they are members of the patient's biological family or part of the healthcare team, the 'professional family'. Caregivers need support to enable them to continue caring; there needs to be a clear sense of integration and 'connectedness' so that care exists in a dynamic framework rather than as something passive which is given by the doctor to the patient.

As the play progresses Davies begins to appreciate his vulnerability, his lack of integration within his environment, and he starts to complain to Mick about the gas stove and his lack of conversation (interaction) with Aston. A further sense of dislocation is temporal: he yearns for a clock and claims 'I mean, if you can't tell what time you're at you don't know where you are'. Elderly patients may become disorientated with respect to time after admission to hospital and this may contribute to their sense of helplessness.

Like Aston's broken monologue, Davies' fractured discursive patterns, and in the whole play, silences and half-sentences show a lack of linguistic polish or connectedness which reflects the intensity of the characters' feelings. In his original programme notes for *The Caretaker* Pinter remarks:

> A character on the stage who can present no convincing argument or information as to his past experience, his present behaviour or his aspirations, nor give a comprehensive analysis of his motives is as legitimate and as worthy of attention as one who, alarmingly, can do all these things. The more acute the experience the less articulate its expression.[13]

Sometimes doctors may refer to patients as 'poor historians' when in fact they are reflecting their own inadequacy in eliciting the concerns of a distressed patient. Patients are often stunned by the news of recurrence of their cancer and temporarily their suffering is mute. It is not possible for them to make sensible decisions about their future care while in this state; they need time and support to adjust to their new situation.

If Aston's inhuman treatment represents the harm caused by active intervention, the ending of the play can be seen to demonstrate how the brothers' failure to care can be equally damaging. Davies cannot find any sense of security within the house, being unable to connect with Aston's trauma and lacking any kind of background that would make him suitable for Mick's mocking 'job offer' of caretaker. Davies, too, has suffered from a persistent lack of care as he drifts from job to job and is given very little external support. Mick perhaps momentarily recognises this lack of care and thus his offer, and subsequent mocking withdrawal, of the job of caretaker is particularly crushing:

> 'How could I have got the wrong man? You're the only man I've spoken to. You're the only man I've told, about my dreams, about my deepest wishes, you're the only one I've told, and I only told you because I understood you were an experienced first-class professional interior and exterior decorator.'

It is clear that Davies does not have the relevant qualifications for such a job, but Mick's feigned shock and labelling of the old man as an 'impostor' is poisonous: he suggests that Davies has tricked him into a form of intimacy, of a human connection where he has shared his dreams. This is precisely the kind of benevolence and respect that both Davies and Aston have been seeking.

Later Davies begins actively to quarrel with Aston who simply says, 'I think it's about time you find somewhere else. I don't think we're hitting it off.' Davies counters by saying he is staying on as caretaker on his brother's orders. After a silence, Aston tells him that he stinks. Davies pathetically stutters 'You ain't . . . you ain't got the right . . .' In the next scene pressure mounts when Mick also tells Davies that he stinks and is 'completely unpredictable'. He then pays him off as caretaker with 'half a dollar'. Davies asks, 'What about me?' only to be met with silence.

Aston enters and Davies starts a desperate bargaining in the forlorn hope that he can stay, even offering to help Aston to build his shed, but Aston simply turns his back and looks out the window. This turning away is an ultimate expression of distancing and a lack of connection. A parallel can be drawn in a clinical situation when patients can feel that they are of little interest when a doctor turns away to read a computer screen or to study the case records during the consultation.

In the end, it is the brothers' silence and inactivity that drives Davies to despair.

The final 11 lines of the play all belong to Davies, and are punctuated by silences from Aston who crucially turns his back for a second time. Davies is left to stew in a mass of fragmented, unfinished sentences that communicate his sense of utter disconnection within his environment, leading to a disturbing and truncated conclusion:

'Listen . . . if I . . . got . . . down . . . if I was to . . . get my papers . . . would
you . . . would you . . . would you let . . . would you . . . if I got down . . .
and got my . . .'
Long silence.
Curtain.

In many ways the balance of power has shifted, since Aston does nothing to
intervene in Davies' plight. Aston has been damaged when forcibly placed in
an institution and given a debased form of 'care'; here he stands by and allows
Davies to be expelled into an uncaring outside world. Both men have sought
to find some form of integration, of connectedness, but the legacy of Aston's
abuse and society's lack of care for Davies turn the men into adversaries in a
competition for the same space. Davies tries to stake his claim to the house but
cannot express himself coherently and must face the future alone. The eviction
of the elderly and frail Davies from the household is a painful example of a
breakdown of mutual care. Davies now faces the unknown and his feelings of
uncertainty are shared by many patients who are discharged prematurely from
hospital without adequate support.

A MODEL OF CARE

Doctors, nurses and students may find difficulties in dealing with their own
emotions when caring for patients at the end of their lives.[12] Such difficulties
may be hard to address in the clinical setting. A study of *The Caretaker* may give
healthcare professionals and students an opportunity to reflect on their own
feelings about end-of-life care. This interprofessional perspective may also help
drama students to gain new insights into Pinter's work.

Some clinical concepts of care can be summarised in the following model
of end-of life care. Elements of this model are explored in more detail in the
rest of the book. The issues raised in *The Caretaker* act as a trigger for reflection.

Teaching and learning about the concept of care benefits from adopting an
interdisciplinary approach. Creating a culture of learning where participants
feel safe to disclose their emotions and fears is fundamental to this approach.
Skilled facilitation and sensitive feedback are also important factors in this type
of experiential learning.[14] These issues are examined in detail in Chapter 10.

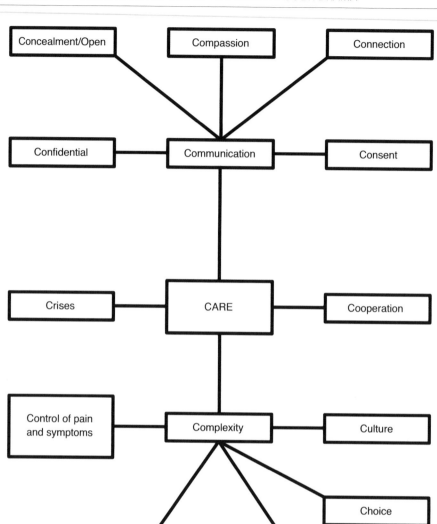

FIGURE 2.2 Model of care at the end of life

CONCLUSION: *THE CARETAKER* AND GOOD END-OF-LIFE CARE

A study of *The Caretaker* emphasises the importance of maintaining a patient's dignity and of fostering realistic hopes for their future care. When Aston remarks of his traumatic experience at the psychiatric hospital, 'I could never quite get it together', he captures not only the essence of the play but also a fundamental anxiety in the context of end-of-life care. In Pinter's play there is a pervasive sense of dislocation and disconnection. The characters seek a sense of coherence; they strive to find a place where they may receive care, where they may feel both validated and valued. The protagonists suffer from both active intervention (Aston's brainwashing) and a dereliction of a duty of care (failure to give continuing shelter to Davies). Patients often describe their suffering as a form of disconnection, of not being themselves, a crisis of identity, or 'not being able to get it together'. Silence can be helpful but also can be a form of deprivation. As we explore in Chapter 7, suffering is difficult to describe precisely because it has a negative quality; something is not as it should be. An important aim of end-of-life care is to facilitate the patient's engagement with their suffering, to allow them time and space to gain a sense of meaning from their life, to regain a sense of connection and to give them the best chance to die in comfort with a sense of completion.[15]

A study of *The Caretaker* can be one way of allowing medical students and doctors to discuss their emotions in a neutral arena which does not threaten their sense of being a 'good doctor'. Doctors need to accept that they are vulnerable and unable to 'do something' in every situation. Simply to listen and to remain with a patient who has unrelieved suffering is a remedy. By studying *The Caretaker* doctors may see that empathy is not simply an attribute that one may possess but is a form of alignment or connection with the other person at an emotional level.

The suffering of the dying is poorly understood and research into this group of patients may be seen as intrusive and ethically inappropriate. As a form of unobtrusive research into the plight of dying patients, a study of *The Caretaker* can teach healthcare professionals much about engaging with suffering.

REFERENCES

1 Peacock DK. *Harold Pinter and the New British Theatre*. London: Greenwood Press; 1997.
2 Somers J. *The Birthday Party*: its origins, receptions, themes and relevance for today. *Cycnos*. 1997; **14**: 7–18.
3 Frank AW. *The Renewal of Generosity*. Chicago: University of Chicago Press; 2004.
4 Calman KC. Quality of life in cancer patients: an hypothesis. *J Med Ethics*. 1984; **10**: 124–7.

5 Slevin ML, Stubbs L, Plant HJ *et al*. Attitudes to chemotherapy: comparing views of patients with cancer with those of doctors, nurses and the general public. *BMJ*. 1990; **300**: 148–60.

6 Munday D, Mather EJ. Informed consent and palliative chemotherapy. *BMJ*. 2008; **337**: 868.

7 Silvestri G, Pritchard R *et al*. Preferences for chemotherapy in patients with advanced non small cell lung cancer; descriptive study based on scripted interviews. *BMJ*. 1998; **17**: 771–5.

8 Audrey S, Abel J, Blazeby JM *et al*. What oncologists tell patients about survival benefits of palliative chemotherapy and implications for informed consent: qualitative study. *BMJ*. 2008; **337**: 752.

9 The A-M, Hak T, Koeter G *et al*. Collusion in doctor–patient communication about imminent death: an ethnographic study.' *BMJ*. 2000; **321**: 1376–81.

10 National Confidential Enquiry into Patient Outcome and Death. *Systemic Anti-Cancer Therapy: for better, for worse?* 2008. Available online at: www.ncepod.org.uk/2008report 3/Downloads/SACT_summary.pdf (accessed 25 April 2010).

11 Connelly JE. The avoidance of human suffering. *Perspect Biol Med*. 2000; **52**: 381–91.

12 Chochinov HM. Dignity and the essence of medicine: the ABC and D of dignity-conserving care. *BMJ*. 2007; **335**: 184–7.

13 Pinter H. Writing for theatre. In: Osborne J, editor. *Plays One*. London: Faber & Faber; 1991.

14 Jeffrey D, editor. *Teaching Palliative Care: a practical guide*. Oxford: Radcliffe Medical Press; 2002.

15 George R. Suffering and healing: our core business. *Palliat Med*. 2009; **23**: 385–7.

CHAPTER 3

Connection: *Journey's End*, RC Sherriff (1928)

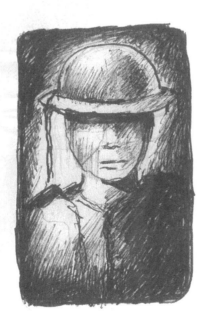

INTRODUCTION

RC Sherriff famously said, 'I meddled in things which man must leave alone,'[1] and *Journey's End* uncompromisingly depicts the chaos of frontline trench warfare, an unpalatable truth to his contemporary audiences who initially found the play distasteful. The chaos may be mirrored, to an extent, in clinical situations of complexity, confusion, fear and suffering, once graphically described by Schon as 'the swampy lowlands'.[2]

Life-threatening illness is a form of crisis which demands a re-examination of goals, beliefs and values. While it is impossible to eradicate all suffering it is always possible to address suffering by connecting with patients and with their families.

Such connection between the doctor and patient sends a message of support and communicates the desire to understand another's point of view. We would like to explore the notion of connection in this chapter with a particular focus on the connections between the characters in the play (a form of surrogate family) and how this form of family faces and copes – or fails to cope – with the pressures of an extremely challenging environment. In turn we will draw parallels with the doctor–patient relationship in terminal care.

Healthcare professionals need to be aware of their own emotions if they are to give effective psychological and spiritual support to patients and families. Self-awareness necessarily involves connecting with oneself. This connection is a step towards the Socratic imperative 'Know Thyself'. It is by reflecting on our actions and feelings that we become mindful and gain what Socrates calls *phronesis* or practical wisdom.

Since no individual can possibly meet all the needs of the dying patient multidisciplinary teamwork is an essential part of responding to the needs of a patient and their family. While working as part of a team is supportive for healthcare professionals, the constant exposure to death and dying can be emotionally draining. There is a risk that an individual, or even a team, may become stressed and show signs of burnout. Burnout or compassion fatigue may occur when healthcare professionals are overwhelmed by their work and can no longer function effectively. In *Journey's End*, the stresses of life in the front line lead to exhaustion, stress and mental breakdown. In the aftermath of the fighting in the Middle East there is great interest at present in the prevention and management of post-traumatic stress disorder which can be seen as an extreme form of burnout.

Good communication lies at the heart of the doctor–patient relationship, yet there are often times when doctors are silent about difficult emotional problems. Sometimes a problem may become 'the elephant in the room', a massive presence which is nevertheless ignored. In *Journey's End* the soldiers deny the seriousness of their situation in light banter which hides 'the elephant in the room'. Lines of communication and the role of hierarchies involved in care will also be explored in this chapter. Doctors and nurses work in hierarchies of power that can create tensions and problems which affect patient care. These hierarchies are clear in *Journey's End* and reflect some issues that are relevant to the working of the multidisciplinary team in palliative care. There may also be conflicts between the patient's biological family and the professional 'family' providing the care.

PLAY SYNOPSIS

Journey's End depicts the experience of a young, naive and idealistic soldier Raleigh who is thrust into the midst of trench life in the First World War. The play opens with Hardy, a captain, being relieved of his position by Lieutenant Osborne. Hardy expresses jocular concern about Captain Stanhope (who is due to arrive in the trenches) and Stanhope's drink problem, but Osborne backs Stanhope and is quick to defend him. We are introduced to Private Mason, who is supposed to be the cook but is somewhat lackadaisical, and the Second Lieutenant Trotter. In these opening stages we also meet the naive and idealistic young soldier who waits for the arrival of Stanhope, with some anticipation: Stanhope was a high achiever and charismatic sportsman at the school they both attended. Raleigh has specifically requested to join Stanhope's company, which irritates Stanhope, who is somewhat different from Raleigh's memory, being a disillusioned, traumatised individual with a clearly burgeoning alcohol problem.

Through the course of the play we watch how the company of soldiers attempt to negotiate their fragile situation with forced camaraderie, relying on the scant comfort of poor-quality food and taking refuge in drink. Stanhope finds himself an unwilling mentor to Raleigh, and the latter, to begin with, maintains a sense of loyalty to his former schoolmate. We learn that Stanhope is in a relationship with Madge, Raleigh's sister, and at the end of Act 1 he confides that he is worried Raleigh will write to her and inform her of Stanhope's drinking. Stanhope tells Osborne that he intends to censor any letters that Raleigh sends home and, drunk, is put into bed by his lieutenant.

Act 2 develops the sense of tedium and anxiety that the men experience and the difference in world-view between Raleigh's youthful optimism and Osborne's weariness of the war. Osborne and Raleigh discuss the school they attended and Osborne reveals that he is tired of the war and talks about the absurdity of two countries being engaged in a pointless war of attrition. The sense of foreboding is increased as Stanhope indicates an attack is imminent and that the trench defences need to be repaired. Stanhope steals a letter that Raleigh has been writing to his sister, intent on covering up his own drinking problem, but Raleigh has portrayed Stanhope in a very positive light, making the captain feel guilty.

In the next scene, the men prepare for a daylight raid on the Germans with the aim of capturing and interrogating an enemy soldier. Raleigh is excited and again demonstrates his naivety as he appears unaware of the real danger the mission will involve. Second Lieutenant Hibbert complains of neuralgia in his eye and becomes hysterical as he tells Stanhope he would rather risk being shot as a deserter than go on the forthcoming mission. Stanhope confides in Hibbert that he himself is scared, and this seems to calm Hibbert as they agree to 'stick it together'.

Stanhope then tries to rally the men for the raid, and is angered when Osborne gives him his ring in case he shouldn't return alive. Stanhope insists that the mission will be a success. The raid takes place, and Osborne is killed in the process. A traumatised Raleigh returns, disillusioned with the war and horrified at the death of the lieutenant. The relationship between Raleigh and Stanhope starts to break down, as Raleigh refuses to eat with the senior officers and the young man expresses anger that his commanders have a form of 'celebration' without recognising that Osborne has died.

The German attack on the trench finally takes place, and Raleigh is badly wounded by a shell that has broken his spine. Stanhope puts Raleigh into Osborne's bed and tries to soothe him and comfort him by bringing the candle to his bedside. Raleigh dies, and Stanhope is summoned away just before a German bomb brings the entire trench down and entombs Raleigh.

MODERN INTERPRETATIONS

While we might find some of the language in *Journey's End* dated, the play remains not only a powerful and timely reminder of the dehumanising effects of war but also a testament to the resilience of people placed in the most challenging situations.

Lyn Gardner writes of the 2011 Richmond Theatre production:

> RC Sherriff's account of life in the trenches shortly before a German offen-
> sive could be a creaky old war horse of a drama, with its talk of decent public
> school types, and times being 'topping'. The fact it remains profoundly
> moving, and a terrific old-fashioned treat, is testament to David Grindley's
> scrupulous production, and that Sherriff's play, written in the 1920s and
> based on his own experience, comes straight from the heart.[3]

As the recent tenth anniversary of 9/11 indicates, and after the London atrocities in 2005, we are reminded that we are never far from violent disruption.
Sherriff's juxtaposition of what appears to be a mundane and ordinary social
framework (conversations about food, school days) with the horrors of war
has an echo in Caroline Wyatt's recent description of the gym at an army rehabilitation centre:

> Go to Headley Court rehabilitation centre, or to the recently opened
> Tedworth House recovery centre, and the human impact of a decade of war
> in Afghanistan is all too clear. As you watch an early-morning physical train-
> ing session in the gym at Tedworth House in Wiltshire, what you notice first
> is the intense focus and fierce concentration of the fit young men riding
> exercise bikes, or pushing up weights as if their lives depended on it. Only
> gradually do you register their missing limbs, and the still livid scars that
> shrapnel and debris from a bomb blew deep into their flesh.[4]

In Chapter 7, we will look at Sarah Kane's harrowing and brutal play *Blasted*
where two 'ordinary' individuals, Cate and Ian, are suddenly taken out of the
safety and comfort of a luxury hotel and plunged into a bitter civil war. Yet, for
Cate and Ian, this plunge into a life-threatening situation is utterly unexpected,
whereas the soldiers in *Journey's End* are aware that danger is always present,
and the possibility of a fatal bomb strike is a realistic one. *Blasted* forcefully
reminds us that theatre has the facility to explore how our ontological security
can be unexpectedly shattered in the same way as a diagnosis of terminal illness can represent a personal crisis for the patient.

We wish to explore the connections between the characters in *Journey's End* and consider how these form support systems which are healthy and positive for the characters as well as forms of apparent 'support' that are damaging and represent negative patterns in both the context of the play and in terminal care.

CLINICAL CONTEXT

When a patient has a life-threatening diagnosis it may be difficult for the doctor to find an appropriate time to ascertain the patient's wishes for care at the end of their life. In general conversation, to talk about death is often regarded as being morbid, as witnessed by many people's reluctance to make a will. When the future is more unpredictable, as in the case of patients with cardiac or respiratory failure, it is often harder to know when to broach the subject of the patient's hopes and fears for their future. However, patients need to have an opportunity to talk about end-of-life concerns even though it may be distressing for them. Whether they do get this chance largely depends upon whether they have a doctor who is compassionate, with an understanding of their predicament. Such a doctor will perceive that the patient is worried and will 'connect' with the patient. Doctors and patients have a common purpose and connect when addressing emotional problems during the passage of the illness. Connection involves kindness, empathy and compassion and acknowledges both the dignity of the other person and a shared humanity. Unfortunately, such 'soft' virtues are often neglected in health organisations which prefer to focus on targets and measurable outcomes and so overlook support for doctors who may be stressed by their work. Consequently, healthcare professionals may develop avoidance tactics, such as appearing busy, ignoring emotional cues or focusing on technical aspects of care. Such rituals do not serve the patient's real needs and furthermore lead to feelings of failure, frustration and grief in the doctor and ultimately to the syndrome of burnout.

The challenge in connecting with patients is to learn to be open with another person and to accept vulnerability without avoidance tactics or trying to 'fix it'. Many doctors underestimate the value of simply being present, remaining silent, and allowing patients to express emotions.

EMPATHY

Empathy is the ability to appreciate the emotions and feelings of others and to develop a connection with them. Empathy enables doctors to understand the inner experience of patients, to communicate this understanding, and to respond in a therapeutic way. It is both the recognition and acknowledgement of the other's individuality and humanity.[5] Guidance from the General Medical Council (GMC) refers to empathy and describes it as one of the qualities of a good doctor.[6] Compassion, empathy and caring are central to the doctor–patient relationship. One of the justifications for including a study of the humanities in medical education is to foster empathy in medical students. There is a danger that with the increasing bureaucracy in medical education idealism and empathy may dwindle.[5]

Too much emotional involvement may also be harmful, so tension exists for the doctor or nurse between maintaining objectivity and establishing empathy. In some situations, such as emergency surgery, effective practice depends on the surgeon being able to distance herself from the subjective world of the patient. However, there is a danger that with technological advances and increasing workloads doctors become inappropriately distant from the patient in situations of chronic illness and end-of-life care and consequently no longer perceive themselves as healers but as technicians.[7] The high moral standards demanded of doctors by the GMC and society risk creating feelings of inferiority in patients. Doctors may be viewed as terribly busy and, in exceeding the requirements of duty, deserving of the patient's gratitude.

It is worrying that some research suggests that the ability to empathise with the patient declines during medical school and clinical training.[8] A number of stresses, from harassment to humiliation, may cause a decline in empathy. The study found that idealism among medical students dropped when they were confronted by clinical situations. At this time their focus switched to an interest in technology and objectivity rather than empathy and the 'softer' virtues of compassion and altruism.[8] Other factors which were found to cause stress to doctors and threaten empathy and connection with patients included a lack of social peer support, a high workload, a short duration of patient stay and a lack of positive role models.[8]

TEAM-WORKING

Case history: Charlie

Charlie has advanced pancreatic cancer at the time of diagnosis. Charlie's 'elephant in the room' is his terminal diagnosis and short prognosis. He asks his doctors not to tell his wife Fiona about the seriousness of his situation. His GP feels bound by a duty of confidentiality so all she can do is to try to point out to Charlie the sad consequences of collusion.

Instead of having a chance to be close, the 'elephant in the room' causes a breach in Charlie and Fiona's marriage. The consequence of Charlie's well-meaning but misguided need to protect Fiona is that she is torn by guilt and becomes clinically depressed.

Journey's End contrasts the outlook and behaviour of the novice Raleigh and that of the experienced officer Stanhope, the expert. Doctors develop differing patterns of learning as they gain clinical experience. Johns compares the novice practitioner with the expert.[9] The novice tends to adopt linear thinking in his action, seeing the various aspects of the patient's case as separate problems. On the other hand, the expert, or experienced physician, behaves in a more intuitive fashion, seeing a wider perspective and taking a holistic view of the patient and family. The novice distancing himself from the situation relies on external authorities, believing there must be a 'right answer'. The expert acknowledges his own role in the situation and places reliance on his internal authority. Perhaps the hallmark of the expert is their ability to accept and tolerate uncertainty. The beginner acts by applying knowledge, while the expert uses a reflective intuitive response which is a way of describing wisdom.[9]

On arrival at the front, the newcomer Raleigh says, 'It's – it's not exactly what I thought. It's just this – this quiet that seems so funny.' And later:

> RALEIGH: It seems uncanny. It makes me feel we're – we're all just waiting for something.
>
> OSBORNE: We are, generally, just waiting for something. When anything happens, it happens quickly. Then we just start waiting again.

For some dying patients the last period of their life can be filled with meaning, but for others, unfortunately, it can seem that life is just a boring wait for death. Palliative care teams aim to restore realistic hope by planning achievable goals and to help the patient discover meaning and purpose. Working in multi-disciplinary teams may cause stresses which can threaten effective teamwork: interprofessional rivalries, leadership difficulties, poor communication and unrealistic expectations of others. Interprofessional power sharing is not always straightforward and this can have a detrimental effect on patient care.

Charlie is helped at home by the primary care team, his GP, the community nurses and home care assistants to provide personal care. The GP feels uncertain that Charlie's pain is optimally controlled. She suggests to the district nurse that specialist Macmillan nurse input might be helpful. The district nurse feels undermined and so replies, 'I don't think they can contribute anything at this stage.'

There can be a temptation for individuals working in the team to be the 'special person' for the patient. This selfish emotion can result in patients receiving sub-optimal care as other team members who could contribute helpfully are effectively blocked from making a contribution.

For healthcare professionals to be aware of the difficulties of teamwork is to counter some of the difficulties of working together. Successive NHS reorganisations which encourage a culture of competition are challenging to teams who are endeavouring to work in a collaborative way. Continuity of care, which is an integral part of a connected approach, is much harder to achieve in a modern setting. In palliative care professional roles overlap and this may lead to interprofessional disputes over the care of a patient. There may be a lack of understanding of the skills of other team members which leads to unrealistic expectations. A community nurse may not understand why a specialist Macmillan nurse does not carry out 'hands-on' care. It may be that nurses seem to work harder at their relationships with doctors than doctors do with nurses. Doctors do not seem to negotiate care and relationships in the same way as nurses do. This may reflect the differences in power between the two professions.[10] Doctors may perceive a nurse's suggestion about prescribing as a criticism of their skills. When such difficulties arise doctors and nurses may direct care to maintain their professional boundaries to the detriment of the patient and their family. Respecting the autonomy of fellow professionals in different disciplines breaks down these boundaries and creates a team spirit conducive to achieving the aims of palliative care.

In the play the first hint of team rivalry occurs in Act 1 when Hardy and

Osborne are discussing Stanhope's drinking. Hardy suggests that Osborne ought to be commanding the company.

> OSBORNE: He was out here before I joined up. His experience alone makes him worth a dozen people like me.
>
> HARDY: You know as well as I do, you ought to be in command.

In hospitals, consultants are generally regarded as leaders of the clinical teams. In some cases these doctors may have power and a certain control over nursing work. This is an outdated model based on a paternalistic approach and where nurses may face a conflict as their loyalties are divided between the doctor, patient, nurse colleagues and their manager.

In the trenches, Stanhope expects his fellow officers to eat together and not with the lower ranks. He confronts Raleigh who had some bread and cheese with the men.

> STANHOPE: Are you telling me – you've been feeding with the men?
>
> RALEIGH: Well, Sergeant Baker suggested.
>
> STANHOPE: So you take your orders from Sergeant Baker, do you?

These firm hierarchies exist in the army but are not appropriate in multiprofessional healthcare teams. Verghese comments poignantly on the loneliness of a senior doctor:

> Despite all our grand societies, memberships, fellowships, speciality colleges, each with its annual dues and certificates and ceremonials, we are horribly alone. The doctor's world is one where our own feelings – particularly those of pain and hurt – are not easily expressed, even though patients are encouraged to express theirs. We trust our colleagues, we show propriety and reciprocity, we have scientific knowledge, we learn empathy, but we rarely expose our own emotions.[11]

The vital 'care' component of nursing is difficult to measure and so becomes vulnerable to an organisation driven by market forces. These forces operating in the NHS threaten the invisible components of holistic care of dying patients.

Nurses and young doctors may now feel guilty for spending time with patients. Yet by carrying out such personal care of patients they are emotionally closer to them and more aware of their wider needs. Doctors need to listen to this holistic perspective.

The expert medical knowledge of doctors and their access to a wide range of investigations and treatments gives them power over patients. Currently, there is concern about the extent of this power and its focus on 'high-tech' interventions to the detriment of the caring elements of practice.[12] Recent reports on care of the elderly in hospital and in care homes reflect these concerns.[13,14] There is a risk that doctors become seen as competent but distanced from the patient's suffering yet retaining the power to prescribe, forbid or even harm. These considerable powers should only be exercised with the patient's free, informed and understood consent. Such informed consent acts as a brake on the power of the doctor.

Another mechanism for limiting the power of doctors over patients can be seen when the nurse acts as an advocate for the patient. Advocacy involves representing the cause of another person to a higher authority. Although in an ideal world advocacy in healthcare would be unnecessary since all healthcare professionals should be acting in the best interests of patients, sometimes doctors may be perceived as being 'too busy to listen', so nurses can help by presenting the patient's view. Difficulties can arise when the doctor misinterprets such advocacy as a personal criticism.

Healthcare professionals from differing disciplines need to work with patients and families in a partnership between the professional and biological families involved in the care of a patient. Mutual trust and respect of each other's expertise facilitate the flourishing of such a partnership. It is illogical to respect patients and yet treat one's colleagues as inferiors simply because they work in a different discipline or may be less experienced. The ethical elements of care are heightened in the last weeks of the patient's life. The process of palliative care can be a time of moral development for both the patient and the many who care for her.

Addressing issues of death and dying can be difficult for everyone: doctors, nurses, patients and their families. If patients are not encouraged to discuss their fears, death becomes the 'elephant in the room', unavoidable, unacknowledged and in some ways taboo.[15]

While at the front two officers avoid talking about the recent deaths of their comrades:

> HARDY: They simply blew us to bits yesterday . . .
>
> OSBORNE: Do much damage?
>
> HARDY: Awful. A dug-out got blown up and came down in the men's tea. Damned annoying.
>
> OSBORNE (lighting his pipe and smoking): I know. There's nothing worse than dirt in your tea.

If the 'elephant' is faced and the patient given the opportunity to discuss their fears then anxieties diminish, realistic planning for the remaining life can proceed and there is a chance for the patient to find meaning.

Towards the end of the play Osborne is about to leave on a dangerous mission. He asks Stanhope to give his watch and a letter to his wife if he is killed on the sortie. Instead of acknowledging that this is a sensible precaution and giving Osborne a chance to say goodbye, Stanhope denies that there is a chance of his being killed.

> OSBORNE: I say, don't think I'm being morbid, or anything like that, but would you mind taking care of these for me?
>
> STANHOPE: Sure. Until you come back old man.
>
> OSBORNE: It's only just in case – if anything should happen, would you send these along to my wife? (He pauses and gives an awkward little laugh).
>
> STANHOPE: You're coming back, old man. Damn it! What on earth should I do without you?
>
> OSBORNE (facing him and laughing): Goodness knows!
>
> STANHOPE: Must have somebody to tuck me up in bed. Well, I'll see you in the sap, before you go. Just have a spot of rum in that coffee.
>
> OSBORNE: Righto.

This false jollity works to ignore the 'elephant in the room' that death is highly probable. Doctors sometime adopt this jocular tone in language such as 'just pop up on the couch, I need to listen to your chest' or 'this is just a small scratch' when attempting to insert an intravenous line. In end-of-life care it might be pretending that a final course of palliative chemotherapy is going to 'control the disease'. The jocular language used to try to obscure the 'elephant in the room' is only one form of coping strategy. We have seen in the previous chapter on *The Caretaker* how the characters rely on particular objects or tasks that affirm their identity and make them feel safe. Aston wants to build his shed and constantly fiddles with an electric plug, perhaps as a way of diffusing the traumatic memories of his ECT treatment. Davies is convinced that once he reaches Sidcup, his 'papers' will establish his 'real' persona. In *Journey's End*, we see a similar phenomenon. Osborne reads sections of *Alice in Wonderland* to Trotter, a childlike fantasy that seems incongruous in the military context. Stanhope clearly relies on alcohol to block out the horrors of war, and the repeated reference by most characters to the mundane details of their food is evidently a way of blocking out the desperate nature of their situation. In our later chapter on *All My Sons* we will see how Joe Keller, a retired successful factory owner, hides his guilty feelings about his past by breezily talking about offering his disgraced former partner a job.

There is, therefore, a problem here in the sense of being 'realistic' about the situation of both the characters and terminally ill patients. Although we must recognise that there must be clarity in communication and no attempt to hide the reality of the situation, we must accept that patients will have different coping strategies. The issue arises here of when a 'coping' strategy may become destructive.

It might be useful here, in this respect, to look in detail at the scene in which the terrified Hibbert desperately tries to avoid taking part in the dangerous raid and admits his vulnerability to Stanhope, indicating that he is thinking of risking being shot as a deserter as he is so afraid. This powerful scene shows the damage that the 'jocularity' has inflicted – far from screening the challenges of conflict it has caused the characters to suppress their true feelings.

Stanhope admits to Hibbert that 'Sometimes I just feel I could lie down on this bed and pretend I was paralysed . . . just lie there till I died . . .'

One may feel for Hibbert in his distress, but also see the compassion that Stanhope displays in revealing that he himself is scared, and that to be scared is not irrational or cowardly but a natural human response to the situation. In this scene we see that the 'elephant in the room' is being acknowledged by the senior officer admitting his vulnerability and the real issue is then negotiated.

COMMUNICATION, SPACE AND THE 'OUTSIDE WORLD'

Sherriff heightens the claustrophobia of the soldiers' quarters not only through using only one room as the setting but by emphasising in the dramatic narrative that communication with those at home was problematic and piecemeal, and letters were censored by senior officers for fear of disclosing military strategy. The men have no privacy either in their correspondence or from each other: another reason why the conversations are mundane. Just as Hibbert is obviously distressed at the possibility of his 'incompetence' being disclosed, Stanhope is terrified at the idea that Raleigh will write to Madge and reveal Stanhope's alcoholic behaviour and inability to cope: when Stanhope finally opens the letter surreptitiously he finds instead that Raleigh has written a very positive appraisal.

It was Florence Nightingale who first emphasised the importance of the physical environment in caring for patients. Privacy is now treated as a human need and can be thought of as a withdrawal from public view or company.[17] Privacy has a number of components: physical aspects include the idea of one's personal space, an invisible space surrounding the person and serving to separate or protect people from one another. Patients may feel an invasion of their personal space by being asked to undress for a clinical examination. Patients feel a lack of privacy in hospital wards which are noisy, and conversations with doctors are shared with other patients behind flimsy screens. Furthermore patients may feel a lack of privacy and space in sleeping in a ward with other patients. Another physical concept is that of territory: the physical space, such as home, where people may feel relaxed and free to question or resist suggestions for treatment. This may be contrasted with the hospital environment where the same person may feel submissive and withdrawn. Territories can be manipulated administratively to ensure compliance and to maintain hospital regimes.

CASE EXAMPLE: MARY

Mary had metastatic breast cancer and had received two courses of chemotherapy, but in spite of this the cancer was spreading to her bones, lungs and liver. She felt tired and was fed up with going to the hospital; the search for a parking space, the long wait to see her doctor and the further waiting for her treatment were getting her down. She talked at home with her Macmillan nurse and told her that she was definitely going to stop having chemotherapy and would tell her consultant that afternoon.

The next day the Macmillan nurse called in to see how Mary had fared at the clinic. To her surprise Mary told her that once she was in the clinic, everyone seemed so busy she did not have the energy to resist the treatment as she did not want to make a fuss. She just went along with having another course of chemotherapy despite the fact that it was making her feel worse.

Psychological privacy is the space which gives people time for reflection and gives permission for patients to limit the information they wish to share. Social aspects of privacy allow patients to be on their own at times if they wish. Seeking a patient's permission to speak to them, simple acts like knocking on a door before entering are small but important signals of respect for a person's privacy. Factual privacy relates to how and when information about a patient is released to others and relates to issues of confidentiality.

In all the plays we explore in this book, we can trace a familiar theme of isolation or feelings of hostility from an 'uncaring' or dangerous outside world. The apparent havens that the characters have found offer no real comfort, from the semi-derelict leaking house in *The Caretaker* to the stifling environment of colonial Africa in Churchill's *Cloud 9*.

COMPASSION

Throughout *Journey's End* the relationship between Stanhope and Raleigh has been volatile, from Stanhope's irritation at Raleigh's initial hero worship to Raleigh's disgust at the 'celebratory' meal that is in fact masking the trauma of Osborne's death. We might argue that at the end of the play, when the wounded Raleigh is comforted by Stanhope who brings a candle nearer his bed, the older man is demonstrating a degree of compassion and a form of closure on the moments of tension and anger between the two men. In Kane's *Blasted* this is realised in an even starker manner, with the character of Cate feeding her blinded and dependent boyfriend.

There are some simple practical steps which facilitate the development of empathy and compassion in end-of-life care. The environment must be conducive for communication. Just as the soldiers crave their own space, a patient may require a quiet setting and a doctor or nurse with time to explore sensitive issues. Eliciting concerns involves asking questions such as, 'How is the illness affecting you and your family?' It also involves exploring the patient's own ideas and feelings: 'How are you coping with this?' The patient should have an opportunity to discuss their view of the future. 'Help me to understand what this is like for you; would you like to talk about your hopes and fears for the future?'

Empathy involves the appreciation and acknowledgement of the suffering of others. The doctor needs to convey to the patient that they matter. An open consultation style, the use of silence and an ability to listen are essential for empathy. The doctor has to appreciate that to understand a patient's experience requires sensitive questioning. Patients will often give doctors cues such as 'I am worried that my wife won't cope with the news', to test whether the doctor is prepared to enter his emotional world and to feel their suffering without apprehension. Looking into the face of another's suffering also compels the doctor to confront their own attitudes to death and dying.

Empathic statements might include acknowledging the patient's feelings: 'This must be difficult for you.' Empathy also involves respecting the patient and affirming their coping strategies. It involves giving the patient a commitment to work together: 'Let's plan the next stage together; what is most important for you?'

With empathy established the conversation can then move on to allow the patient to reveal their resources and to form a plan together.

BURNOUT

Continuity of care is one of the foundations of good communication and is essential in building a trusting relationship between the healthcare professional and the patient and their family. Paradoxically, patients may feel powerless in institutions that were created to help them. Patients may be perceived by politicians as 'problems' rather than seen as individuals who matter.[16] Suffering then can be perceived as a problem of rising financial costs for healthcare. A distance is created between those who make the political decisions and those healthcare professionals at the bedside. The concern for governments is to create policies and there is a risk that doctors can then become merely the agents whose responsibility is to implement the policy; for example, 'only carrying out orders'.[16] Frank talks of how care then becomes an 'allocation' determined by management. This applies both to the doctor in the ward and for a soldier in battle. The conflict for staff occurs because those receiving the orders, or targets, are in the action, while those giving the orders or issuing the targets remain safe at a distance. The doctor or nurse is presented with speaking with the voice of management yet the person in front of them demands their professional time, care and expertise.[16] It is part of the professional's responsibility to speak out in these situations rather than compromising our standards and taking short cuts which cause both the patients and the doctors enormous stress.

Terminally ill patients are vulnerable and may often display strong emotions to which doctors may respond with feelings of their own: powerlessness, grief, or a desire to escape.[16] Doctors have an obligation to be aware of their own emotions and to recognise the way in which they can affect patient care. For instance, a doctor who has a strong urge to 'rescue the patient' may experience a patient's death from advanced cancer as both a personal and a professional failure. If doctors fail to identify their emotions serious consequences may follow; perhaps patients may be subject to inappropriate life-prolonging technologies in situations where active treatments are known to be futile. Or conversely patients may be abandoned as the doctor feels so bad that there is no longer a possibility of cure. In extreme cases the doctor may experience burnout which is characterised by a progressive loss of idealism, compassion, energy and purpose. Burnout results in a failure to care and can be the result of the cumulative exposure to suffering, death and grief.[18] However, it is also interesting to observe that many of the stresses healthcare professionals experience are related to working with difficult colleagues and institutional hierarchies rather than caring for dying patients.[18]

From the outset of the play we are aware that Stanhope is suffering severe stress.

> OSBORNE: He's a long way the best company commander we've got.
>
> HARDY: Oh, he's a good chap, I know. But I never did see a youngster put away the whiskey he does. D'you know, the last time we were out resting at Valennes he came to supper with us and drank a whole bottle in one hour fourteen minutes — we timed him.

Alcohol abuse is a common consequence of prolonged stress and just as his fellow officers 'gaze avert' to avoid this 'elephant', so too in healthcare, doctors and nurses tend to ignore heavy drinking in colleagues provided there is no effect on patient care. Watching others struggle is not a professional way to support colleagues.

> OSBORNE: It rather reminds you of bear baiting-or cock-fighting-to sit and watch a boy drink himself unconscious.

Stanhope not only drinks heavily, he doesn't go home on leave, thus 'sticking it, month in, month out'. His fellow officers try to 'hush it up'. Stanhope says: 'There were only two ways of breaking the strain. One was pretending I was ill – and going home; the other was this (He holds up his glass). Which would you pick Uncle?'

Stanhope wonders if he is becoming mentally ill, but he is reassured:

> OSBORNE: Bit of nerve strain, that's all.
> STANHOPE: You don't think I'm going potty?
> OSBORNE: Oh, Lord, no!

Burnout may cause doctors or nurses to become distant and detached from patients, resulting in increased feelings of guilt. In burnout there is often a reduced self-awareness of one's own physical and emotional needs, leading to a self-destructive pattern of overwork. Other features of burnout can include hyperarousal with disturbed sleep, anger, agitation, avoidance or distancing, not wanting to go to the patient, avoiding thoughts and feelings associated with the patient's suffering and intrusive thoughts and distress.[18]

We have seen how Hibbert breaks down and confesses his fear to Stanhope, who reassures him he has the same feelings.

'Stanhope! I've tried like hell – I swear I have. Ever since I came out here I've hated and loathed it . . .'

Stanhope then admits that he has the same feelings.

Support for professionals can re-establish the reciprocal caring relationship. Professionals need to be able to share their own suffering with their colleagues.

Paradoxically, doctors who engage with patients and are empathic have less burnout than those who try to distance themselves from dying patients.[19] Healthcare staff should appreciate the effectiveness of simply being with patients, allowing them to talk and to express emotions. Doctors need to accept the inherent vulnerability of being human without always trying to sort out a problem. Self-awareness can increase the doctor's resilience and ability to continue to empathise and connect with patients. Reflective practice either by writing or by regular clinical supervision with a mentor may give doctors an opportunity to express their feelings and thereby give them the energy and motivation to continue their work without distancing themselves from patients.

MEIR'S REFLECTIVE MODEL

We have seen that doctors who connect with their patients are less likely to suffer burnout, which is a manifestation of compassion fatigue. Achieving an appropriate balance between emotional connection and objective distancing is vital to prevent burnout. Reflection on one's practice is the key to being able to continue to provide compassionate care. Our model is an adaptation of Meir's Reflective Model to Prevent Burnout.[18]

The doctor at risk of burnout

- Identifies *too strongly* with the patient
- Recent bereavement
- Unresolved fears of their own death
- A prolonged dying
- Uncertainty around prognosis
- Disagreements over the goals of care
- Heavy workload
- Sense of failure in looking after dying patients
- Distancing behaviours
- Alcohol abuse
- Lack of peer support.

Signs or symptoms of burnout?

Signs

- Avoiding patients
- Failure to communicate with others
- Failure to attend to details
- Stressed when seeing patients
- Seeing patients more often than necessary.

Symptoms

- Anger
- Intrusive thoughts
- Sense of failure
- Guilt
- Victimised
- Need to save patient.

Name the emotion

- Acknowledging one's emotions is a vital first step in addressing the problem of burnout.

Take time to reflect

- Step back to gain perspective
- Identify behaviours
- Consider implications
- Reframe: think of alternative strategies
- Plan a different approach.

Consult a trusted colleague or mentor

- Sharing the problem is the professional way to address stress and burnout.

CONCLUSIONS

Patients hope that their doctors will be both competent and compassionate so that they receive care which is both appropriate and humane. In the context of the trusting doctor–patient relationship an exchange of emotions occurs, the patient experiences feelings about the doctor (transference) and the doctor about the patient (countertransference). Doctors can use these emotions to provide more effective care which responds to the patient's real needs. Distressing feelings of sadness, anger or helplessness in doctors may reflect the emotions and feelings of their patients who are about to die. Faced with a suffering patient expressing these emotions the doctor is faced with a choice. Either she can respond with compassion and connect with the patient showing empathy and kindness or she can feel overwhelmed and use distancing tactics to avoid addressing emotions. Patients are often quick to gauge whether the doctor in front of them is one who will connect or one who will walk away. If cues are ignored then the patient's suffering will only be increased by a sense of abandonment. In this situation, when the real issues of approaching death are ignored, some doctors may find it easier to prescribe futile treatments or tests in order to maintain a sense of hope.

The proper response to doctors who are suffering from burnout is not professional detachment but supporting them to reconnect with their patients. Even the word 'professional' creates an expectation of being able to cope and may lead the doctor to become isolated from colleagues. Doctors need encouragement to share their distress with colleagues.

Doctors need to be aware of the risks of the compulsive triad of doubt, responsibility and guilt which can so affect a doctor's personal and professional life. If the doctor is unaware of his own emotional needs he may embark on a self-destructive course of overwork. If doctors can connect with patients and empathise, they tend to feel invigorated rather than depleted and this can protect against burnout. Are some doctors more prone to burnout? McManus *et al.* found that doctors who were most stressed showed higher levels of neuroticism while those with the greatest sense of job satisfaction were those with a deep approach to their learning and had more extrovert personalities.[20] In their study they also found that a workplace climate which was unsupportive correlated strongly with stress burnout and low job satisfaction.[20] Interestingly, doctors reporting a workplace climate which was low in support were also rated lower on the personal scale of agreeableness. It seems that happy doctors are those with a deep approach to learning; that is, they have a need to understand the subject. These doctors tend to be more extrovert and have low neuroticism scores.

Kindness, related to compassion, is also a virtue which shows concern for our fellow human beings. It has, however, acquired negative associations in recent times.[21] What is it about our times that makes kindness seem so dangerous?[22] Perhaps being kind is risky because it exposes our vulnerability and our capacity to identify with others suffering. Autonomy and self-reliance have become the benchmarks of ethics in Western society. Relational aspects of mutual dependency have become almost taboo in our society. Kindness encompasses elements of empathy, generosity and humanity and is one manifestation of humanity's desire to connect. But, sadly, it has now become almost a sign of weakness; a virtue of losers. However, everybody is vulnerable to illness, accident or tragedy. We share vulnerability; it is the medium of contact between us. Phillips comments that the pleasure of kindness is that it connects us with each other; the terror of kindness is it makes us aware of our own and others' vulnerability.[22] Kindness opens us up to the world of other people and it is a bridge between the self and the other. Even the Stoic philosophers, renowned for their strong approach to individuality, had a concept of *okeiosis*, a shared community feeling.

Phillips quotes Winnicott writing in 1970:

> A sign of health in the mind is the ability of one individual to enter imaginatively and accurately into the thoughts and feelings and hopes and fears of another person and also to allow the other person to do the same to us.[22]

Dependence is scorned in our modern society, which, in its competitive approach, breeds unkindness. Real kindness is an opening up to engage with others, a solidarity with human need. In *The Descent of Man*, Darwin argues we are a profoundly social and caring species. Palmer suggests that training young doctors in awareness, compassion and kindness may involve reaching out beyond the electronic portfolio and bringing in the humanities.[23] Reflecting on end-of-life care, she asks, 'Did I hear what really matters most for this person right now? Was I kind?'[23]

Connectedness between humans is encapsulated in the South African philosophy of *Ubuntu*. Archbishop Tutu describes a person with *Ubuntu* as welcoming, hospitable, warm, generous, willing to share. Such people are open and available to others, willing to be vulnerable, affirming of others, do not feel threatened that others are able and good for they have a proper self-assurance that they belong in a greater whole and are thus diminished when others are humiliated, tortured or oppressed.[24]

REFERENCES

1 Sherriff, RC. *Columbia World of Quotations*. New York: Columbia University Press; 1996.
2 Schon DA. *Educating the Reflective Practitioner: toward a new design for teaching and learning in the profession*. San Francisco: Jossey-Bass; 1987.
3 Gardner L. *Journeys End* – review. *The Guardian*. 16 March 2011. Available online at: www.guardian.co.uk/stage/2011/mar/16/journeys-end-review (accessed 10 January 2013).
4 Wyatt C, BBC Defence Correspondent. The cost of Afghanistan for British troops. *BBC News*. 9 October 2011. Available online at: www.bbc.co.uk/news/15212872 (accessed 10 January 2013).
5 Smajdor A, Stockl A, Salter C. The limits of empathy: problems in medical education and practice. *J Med Ethics*. 2011; **37**: 380–3.
6 General Medical Council. *Your Health Matters*. GMC; 2010.
7 Dyer C. NHS recommends doctors apologise when treatment goes wrong. *BMJ*. 2009; **338**: 2002.
8 Neuman M, Edelhauser F, Tauschel T *et al*. Empathy decline and its reasons: a systematic review of studies with medical students and residents. *Acad Med*. 2011; **86**: 996–1009.
9 Johns C. *Becoming a Reflective Practitioner*. New York: John Wiley & Sons; 2004.
10 Walshe C, Todd C, Caress A-L, Chew Graham C. Judgements about fellow professionals and the management of patients receiving palliative care in primary care: a qualitative study. *Br J Gen Pract*. 2008; **58**: 264–72.
11 Verghese A. *The Tennis Partner: a doctor's story of friendship and loss*. New York: Harper Collins; 1998.
12 HRH The Prince of Wales. Integrated health in post modern medicine *J R Soc Med*. Doi:10 1258 (jrsm.2012.12k.095) (accessed 29 December 2012).
13 Holt A. Winterbourne View patients in new care safety alert. Available online at: www.bbc.co.uk/news/uk-20070437 (accessed 30 December 2012).
14 Brimelow A. Division in Stafford over scandal-hit hospital. Available online at: www.bbc.co.uk/health-202222283 (accessed 30 December 2012).
15 Griffe J, Nelson-Martin P, Muchka S. Acknowledging the 'elephant': communications

in palliative care: speaking the unspeakable when death is imminent. *Am J Nurs.* 2004; **104**: 48–57.

16 Frank AW. *The Renewal of Generosity*. Chicago: University of Chicago Press; 2004.

17 Leino-Kilpi H, Valimaki M, Dassen T *et al.* Privacy: a review of the literature. *Int J Nurs Stud.* 2001; **38**: 663–71.

18 Meir DE, Back AL, Morrison RS. The inner life of physicians and care of the seriously ill. *JAMA.* 2001; **286**: 3007–14.

19 Kearney MK, Weininger RB, Vachon MLS *et al.* Self-care of physicians caring for patients at the end of life 'Being Connected . . . A Key to My Survival'. *JAMA.* 2009; **301**: 1155–64.

20 McManus IC, Keeling A, Paice E. Stress burnout and doctors' attitudes to work are determined by personality and learning style. A twelve year longitudinal study of UK medical graduates. *BMC Med.* 2004; **2**: 29. Available online at: www.biomedicentral. com/1741-7015/2/29 (accessed 23 September 2012).

21 Einhorn S. *Art of Being Kind*. London: Sphere; 2006.

22 Phillips A, Taylor B. *On Kindness*. London: Hamish Hamilton; 2009.

23 Palmer E. The kindness of strangers. *BMJ.* 2008; **337**: 877.

24 Tutu D. *No Future without Forgiveness*. New York: Image Doubleday; 2000.

CHAPTER 4

Choice: *Antigone,* Sophocles (441 BC)

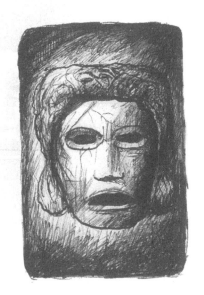

INTRODUCTION

'Life is the sum of all your choices.'

Alfred Camus

What is a choice? Sophocles's audacious and disturbing tragedy *Antigone* explores the social, psychological and cultural factors that may influence or restrict a person's choice as well as exposing the disastrous consequences that may follow a choice (or lack of choice). The play, thought to have been written in 441 BC, is set in Thebes, a self-governing city (*auto nomos*, from which the term autonomy is derived). *Antigone* has a particular resonance today since patients nearing the end of their lives may feel that they have no control over their lives and may fear a loss of both autonomy and dignity. Before we examine a case study which has particular intersections with the issues in *Antigone*, it would be useful to map out the principal tensions relating to choice in Sophocles's play.

ANTIGONE: A PLOT SYNOPSIS

The opening scenes between Antigone and Ismene establish the background to the play. We learn that when the shamed Oedipus was banished from Thebes, Creon became king. Subsequently, Eteocles (Oedipus's son) claimed the throne and exiled his brother Polyneices. Polyneices attacked Thebes, but in the battle the brothers killed each other. Creon declares himself king and gives Eteocles a state funeral. However, he decrees that Polyneices' body must not be buried but left to lie rotting on the battlefield. Such undignified treatment of a body was deeply abhorrent to the Greeks, who believed that a peaceful afterlife in the underworld was dependent on the proper funeral rites being carried out. Creon's decree – if violated – carries the death penalty.

We pick up on the story with Antigone, appalled by Creon's sanction, telling her sister Ismene that she intends to disobey the king, despite her sister's protests. Aware of the danger to herself, Antigone covers the body of her brother with dirt and performs the burial rites. But as she does so, she is caught by the guards who take her to Creon. The king incarcerates both Antigone and her sister Ismene – who took no part in the burial rite. Creon then sentences Antigone to be sealed in a cave to starve to death but releases Ismene. Creon's son, Haemon, who is engaged to Antigone, pleads for her life. Creon refuses his pleas and Haemon leaves, threatening to take his own life.

Tiresias, a blind seer, warns Creon that the gods are angry with him for his disgraceful treatment of Polyneices' body. At first Creon mocks him until the Chorus remind him of the prophet's wisdom. Creon rushes out in an attempt to make amends; he buries the body of Polyneices then goes to the cave to release Antigone. Too late, he discovers Antigone has hanged herself and Haemon is holding her body, distraught with grief. Haemon then plunges a sword into his own body and kills himself in front of his father.

Creon returns to Thebes shattered by his son's suicide. He discovers that his wife Eurydice has also killed herself after learning of her son's death. She curses Creon with her dying breath. Creon finally displays a measure of understanding that he has gained through the bloody consequences of his uncompromising law.

MODERN INTERPRETATIONS OF *ANTIGONE*

Antigone is one of the most frequently performed Greek tragedies and there have been many modern reworkings of Sophocles's narrative to locate the play within different contexts and discourses, such as gender and postcolonial. In a recent article in *The Guardian* newspaper, Charlotte Higgins called Antigone 'a standard-bearer for courage in the face of brutish (male) authority'[1] while Claire Brennan points out that the character has been seen as a 'proto-feminist'.[2] From a sociological perspective there appears to be a central duality, as Ince surmises:

> it is a question of one moral law (honour the dead, honour one's family – two laws coincide) being upheld by Antigone and opposed to another moral law, symbolized by Creon (duty to the state). Antigone's case is stronger than Creon's because there is a true identification between her and the moral law she upholds, whereas Creon, though superficially standing for duty to the state, is really using the moral law he upholds in order to assert his own will. He is the moral law of obedience to the state gone wild: he is a tyrant.[3]

This interpretation of the play is common but is problematic in simplifying the play to a clash of two ideologies; more recent manifestations of the play have teased out some of the complexities of the moral and ethical problems within the text as well as finding new topicalities.

Jean Anouilh's *Antigone* (1943) boldly transfers the action to Nazi-occupied France to explore the intensely sensitive issue of French collaboration with the Nazis. Creon and Antigone appear as still more ambiguous – Antigone is at first forgiven by Creon, but she herself demands that the law is followed. In Athol Fugard's *The Island* (1973) two black political prisoners, on Robben Island,

John and Winston, prepare an 'amateur' production of *Antigone* to show to their fellow convicts, and through the course of the rehearsal they reveal symmetries between their own situation and Antigone's. But Fugard's play also uses the content of *Antigone* to expose interpersonal tensions between the two prisoners, whose futures seem to be very different: John is soon to be released while Winston must continue his sentence. The rehearsal process acts as a catalyst for their arguments: arguments that interrogate the notions of autonomy and freedom. In 2004, Glyn Cannon's *Gone* at the Edinburgh Pleasance presented Sophocles's play in the context of a Britain disillusioned by the Iraq war. The moral dilemmas of *Antigone* are played out by smooth Blairite politicians, with Polyneices' body hidden in a filing cabinet.

The enduring appeal of *Antigone*, then, arguably lies in its universal applicability. Anouilh, Fugard and Cannon all locate Sophocles's play within a particular contemporary political situation to examine issues of personal choice. Yet when we consider the play in the context of end-of-life care, dilemmas presented in *Antigone* can offer some compelling perspectives on personal and social pressures on patients, their families and the medical team. These pressures and tensions relate primarily to the notion of choice.

In *Antigone*, Sophocles explores choice with particular emphasis on issues of individual autonomy, dignity and justice. He describes the actions of a woman caught between her personal moral beliefs and a public morality dictated by Creon's law. These themes are of central importance in the care of patients at the end of life. Sophocles's play is particularly accessible for us today as the moral debate takes place in front of our eyes. The Chorus plays the roles of mediator and counsel, as well as summarising the key developments in the plot and their implications. But there is also an essential humanity to the Chorus, which allows us to engage and empathise with the tragic events as they unfold:

> The Chorus rejoiced in the triumph of good; it wailed aloud its grief, and sympathised with the woe of the puppets of the gods. It entered deeply into the interest of their fortunes and misfortunes, yet it stood apart, outside of triumph and failure. [...] No gladness dragged it into the actual action on the stage, and no catastrophe overwhelmed it, except in storm of sympathetic pain. It was the ideal spectator, the soul being purged, as Aristotle

expressed it, by Pity and Fear, flinging its song and its cry among the passions and the pain of others. It was the 'Vox Humana' amid the storm and thunder of the gods.[4]

By exploring the text to tease out moral issues we too are involved in the discussion and negotiations as well as feeling the pain of the characters.

A CASE HISTORY: MARTHA'S STORY

A case history can illustrate how the moral issues in *Antigone* are relevant to the care of a dying patient.

Martha, a 62-year-old retired teacher, was widowed two years ago. Her husband Ken died suddenly at home with a massive haemorrhage from a lung cancer. Martha has two children: Stephen, a journalist living in New York, and Natalie who is married with a 15-year-old daughter, Tamsin, who live locally.

Nine months ago Martha felt depressed and lost weight, symptoms which her general practitioner thought were due to her grief. However, after three months she was admitted to hospital and found to have advanced pancreatic cancer for which there was no active treatment.

At present Martha is jaundiced and confined to her home where she spends most of the time in bed or sitting in a chair. One afternoon when her GP, Dr Heather Brown, visits Martha asks, 'Doctor, can you help me to die, please?'

Dr Brown is faced with a serious ethical dilemma. She knows that Martha understands that she is going to die in the near future and is making a choice to hasten her death. On one hand, Martha wants to have the option to end her life, without distress at a time of her choosing. On the other hand, hastening death is illegal, may damage the trust patients have in doctors and may put vulnerable people in society at risk.

These thoughts are in Dr Brown's mind as she asks Martha for the reasons behind her choice. Martha reflects on Ken's traumatic death, and admits that she has a horror of becoming incontinent and being a burden to Natalie. Martha asks, 'What is the point of going through a great deal of suffering if my life could be ended peacefully now?'

The issues raised in this case are in part a clash between private and public morality and between the principles of autonomy, justice and non-maleficence.

While Dr Brown may have great sympathy for Martha's request, complying with it conflicts with her duty to other vulnerable patients whose safety might be jeopardised if doctors were permitted to assist in the killing of patients. Doctors and nurses may feel tremendous compassion and sympathy for the plight of a patient who is suffering and who is pleading to have their life ended. However, doctors know that any erosion of their duty not to kill would be disastrous for the relationship of trust which is so essential if doctors and other healthcare professionals are to address suffering. The highly visible media debate on the legalisation of physician-assisted suicide (PAS) can also represent an added pressure on the patient. Typically, the public debate focuses on an articulate, educated individual who advances a pro-PAS argument related to their own medical circumstances. We will explore this social phenomenon later in the chapter.

Palliative care aims to maximise patient autonomy by empowering patients to make choices and to be involved in decisions which affect their care. Philosophers offer a variety of definitions of autonomy, each emphasising a number of different concepts which make up autonomy. For some it means individuality, valuing elements such as choice, whereas others see it as a relational concept which takes into account the needs of others. For instance, we may contrast Gillon's definition, 'Autonomy is the capacity to think, decide and act on the basis of such thought and decision, freely and independently',[5] with that of Dworkin, who states:

> Autonomy is the capacity of persons to reflect critically upon their preferences, desires and wishes and the capacity to accept or attempt to change these in the light of higher-order preferences and values. By exercising such capacity persons define their nature, give meaning and coherence to their lives and take responsibility for the kind of person they are.[6]

Gillon stresses rationality and choice while Dworkin's definition implies that independence and autonomy differ; emphasising self-reflection and the ability to give up a personal choice for a greater good for the majority. Autonomy here is much more than selfishness.

It is important to note that the political description of autonomy for self-governing city states in Ancient Greece is quite different from contemporary understandings of individual autonomy.[7] Kant does not describe individuals as autonomous but outlines law-like principles that could be adopted by all, for instance, the prohibition of taking an innocent life. For Kant the critical issue is that people must never be treated as means to an end but rather must be considered as ends in themselves. This may be contrasted with heteronomous principles like Creon's decree forbidding the funeral of Polyneices, which are adopted by those who defer to some power.[7]

In the first scene Antigone asks her sister Ismene to help her bury her brother Polyneices in spite of the fact that Creon has decreed that anyone who attempts to bury him will die.

'Will you lift up his body with these bare hands and lower it with me?'

Ismene is shocked and in her refusal reminds Antigone that they are only women and cannot break the law:

'Remember we are women, we're not born to contend with men. . . . I must obey the ones who stand in power.'

Antigone does not try to persuade her sister but explains that her duty lies with her personal responsibility to her dead brother, not to Creon's law. Thus there is a clash between her personal morality based on the universal moral laws of the gods and the heteronomous law of Creon.

'Do as you like, dishonour the laws the gods hold in honour.'

In *Antigone* the individual autonomy of Antigone provides a stark clash; she has a personal moral intuition of her duty to her dead brother and so feels justified in breaking Creon's law. In Martha's case she is putting forward an argument for the right for a dying patient to choose the timing and manner of her death and thus to defy the law.

Perhaps we instinctively assume that Antigone was right to defy Creon, but it is possible to take Creon's view that to flout the law is to undermine the security of the state. In some cases friends and relatives have taken terminally ill patients from the UK to Switzerland, where assisted suicide is permitted, thus getting round the UK law. Some of these tragic cases have fuelled the campaign to change the law in the UK to permit assisted suicide and euthanasia.

The primacy of autonomy which goes beyond its Kantian origins has become an accepted part of modern practical ethics. The wrongness of killing in part rests on the fact that to deprive someone of life is to deprive them of their autonomy. However, the individual view of autonomy may suggest that if a person wished their life to be ended by euthanasia or assisted suicide, respect for autonomy would require the doctor to comply with their wishes.

However, as we have seen, the concept of the autonomous person involves more than just the capacity to act on particular choices but extends to include a reflective element which includes a sense of responsibility for the effect of one's choices on the autonomy of others.

Good end-of-life care attempts to empower patients to have as much control as possible, but this raises a question of the limits of autonomy. At what point do issues of justice override the individual's wishes? For when autonomy is taken to be the most important ethical principle there is little discussion of justice – of the needs of others. Rationality may be transiently impaired as one approaches death. How much rationality does a patient need before they are respected as an autonomous individual? A narrow view of autonomy is to see it as self-rule; that is, the ability to choose when and how to die.

A number of considerations arise with Martha's story: for instance, she may be depressed. It is often assumed that all dying patients are depressed and there is not much one can do about it. However, clinical depression is different from the natural sadness that accompanies any form of loss, including dying. Clinical depression can often be successfully treated and patients who recover may change their minds and make different choices about their care. Martha's death affects her family; her son Stephen needs time to travel from New York to see his mother before she dies. Tamsin wants to talk over her choice of A levels with her much loved grandmother. Patients often fear being a burden to their families but once they appreciate how much they can still contribute to others their lives can become meaningful to themselves once more.

A patient's autonomy may be respected in a number of different ways in a clinical setting; by telling the truth, preserving confidentiality and by seeking the patient's informed consent to any proposed medical intervention. There is nothing in the principle of respect for autonomy which requires the doctor to comply with every wish the patient may make. A broad ethical view of autonomy should take account of our essential dependency on others. Death and dying necessarily involves others: family, friends and the wider society. In expressing autonomy an individual gives meaning to their life. This interdependency is particularly evident in Sophocles's play. While we might champion Antigone's sentiment, might we also take issue with the *manner* in which she makes her choice? Can we lay the blame for Haemon's and Eurydice's deaths on Creon's shoulders? Did Antigone consider the shockwaves that her actions would create with full knowledge of the dreadful power of the law?

Particular difficulties arise around considering the consequences of the choice for euthanasia or PAS. In Holland where these practices are legal there is concern that some patients have euthanasia without giving consent.[8] Standards of end-of-life care may not be as high in countries where euthanasia is legal. In Holland, for example, palliative care is not a recognised medical speciality.

Dignity is a concept which is difficult to define. For some people dignity at the end of life means avoiding physical interventions such as tubes and catheters, the absence of pain, not being a burden to others and retaining control over one's body and one's decisions. For some the desire for a dignified death prompts a request for euthanasia or assisted suicide. The Voluntary Euthanasia Society was set up in 1935 and campaigned for the legalisation of euthanasia and assisted suicide. It changed its name to Dignity in Dying in 2006. The Swiss clinic which carries out assisted suicide is known as Dignitas. These uses of the word 'dignity' make an assumption that to die by assisted suicide or euthanasia is to guarantee a dignified death and that to die in another way is somehow undignified. However, a study from the Netherlands revealed that up to 14% of cases of euthanasia or assisted suicide were complicated by problems, such as failure of death, vomiting and muscle twitching.[9]

An individual's dignity can persist after death, as in *Antigone*: the neglect of Polyneice's corpse insults his memory and his family and shocks Theban society. Different senses of dignity are in general use; for example, we attribute dignity by awarding honours such as creating a peerage. However, there is a different sense in which dignity refers to the intrinsic value which all humans possess simply by virtue of the fact that they are human beings; not by virtue of any social standing, or any particular set of talents, skills or powers. Kant's view of intrinsic dignity is summarised in his 'categorical imperative': 'Act in such a way that you treat humanity, whether in your own person or in the person of another, always at the same time as an end and never simply as a means.'[7]

Taylor extends dignity into a sense of 'authenticity', as being true to oneself.

> Only if I exist in a world in which history, or the demands of nature, or the needs of my fellow human beings, or the duties of citizenship, or the call of

God, or something else of this order *matters* crucially, can I define an identity for myself that is not trivial.[10]

This sense of dignity applies to Antigone, who is taking her stand on the basis of her personal conviction of her duty to bury her dead brother and to honour his corpse. It is interesting that the concept of dignity applies to a human corpse; not only does the human body have intrinsic dignity after death but the act of carrying out the funeral rites honours the society and is itself dignified.

Illness and injury can mount an assault on the dignity of human beings that can be overwhelming, so that the person or others may feel he or she has lost all human dignity and, therefore, all moral worth or value. However, as much as intrinsic dignity may be threatened it cannot be lost.

Dignity means that the value of the human is expressed in the ability to stand up to such assaults with courage, humility, acceptance of the finitude of human life, 'nobility and even love'. To kill oneself in the face of death or to ask to be killed, in this view, is precisely the opposite of what it means to face death with dignity.[11]

Martha's request, 'Please, help me to die', may be a way of seeking affirmation from Dr Brown that her life is still important, that she matters. Chochinov's work clearly shows that the attitude of doctors and nurses has a profound effect on the patient's sense of their own dignity.[12] If a doctor is unaware of the possibilities of palliative care or is unable to engage with the patient's suffering in a helpful way, she may feel that hastening the death of the patient is the only way out. A situation where dying is prolonged is particularly difficult for relatives and healthcare professionals even though the patient may be unconscious and not suffering.

'It is not the expression of rationality that makes us human, but our belonging to a kind that is capable of rationality that makes us human.' A sick individual is a member of humankind and, as such, has the intrinsic value we call dignity. 'The plight of the sick has little instrumental value, rarely serving the purposes, beliefs, desires, interests, or expectations of any of us as individuals. Rather, it is because of the intrinsic value of the sick that healthcare professionals serve them.'[11]

Sulmasy says:

The argument from intrinsic dignity suggests that the fundamental basis for the duty to build up the dignity of sick human beings – the root of any motivation to attribute dignity to them – is the intrinsic value of the human, the value human beings have by virtue of being the kinds of things that they are.[11]

Assisted dying, in this view, undermines 'the fundamental basis of morality itself – respect for intrinsic dignity'. The fundamental moral issue is to do with intending to hasten a death, which is to aim at killing human life. It makes sense to say that to adopt this aim is to discount the possibility of any intrinsic worth (or dignity) to human life.

There are other moral reasons to object to assisted dying that include the value of care, which is an expression of human dignity. Also there is a need to listen to clinical instincts, intuitions, principles and practices. From a broad perspective it seems there is the need to maintain the cornerstone of civil law: a prohibition on intentional killing of the innocent.

THE RELATIONSHIP BETWEEN CHOICE AND INFORMED CONSENT

In order to explore choice and informed consent, let us first look in more detail at the choices that face the characters in *Antigone*. The first scene shows us the effect that one choice (Antigone's decision to bury Polyneices) has had on the relationship between the protagonist and her sister. Before Antigone can act on her decision, she tries to enlist the help of her sister in the task: 'Consider if thou wilt share the toil and the deed.' Ismene, in anguish at the request, desperately tries to remind Antigone of the implications of flouting the law:

'Ah me! think, sister, how our father perished, amid hate and scorn, when sins bared by his own search had moved him to strike both eyes with self-blinding hand; then the mother wife, two names in one, with twisted noose did despite unto her life; and last, our two brothers in one day, – each shedding, hapless one, a kinsman's blood, – wrought out with mutual hands their common doom. And now we in turn – we two left all alone think how we shall perish, more miserably than all the rest, if, in defiance of the law, we brave a king's decree or his powers. Nay, we must remember, first, that we were born women, as who should not strive with men; next, that we are ruled of the stronger, so that we must obey in these things, and in things yet sorer. I, therefore, asking the Spirits Infernal to pardon, seeing that force is put on me herein, will hearken to our rulers for 'tis witless to be over busy.'

Ismene's prescience is timely here, and in effect she emphasises that one's actions, though noble in spirit, can have calamitous consequences: in effect, Antigone's choice may well drive others to their own deaths. We may also observe how Ismene effectively highlights the gender inequality and assumption that is a cornerstone of Ancient Greek society. In Chapter 8 on Caryl Churchill's *Cloud 9* we will return to this theme and explore how imposed 'roles' can create psychological distress.

Patient choice is central to the political agenda for the NHS but does not sit comfortably with its ethos. Currently, there is a political belief that choice in itself is beneficial to patients and granting choice improves care. Traditionally, choice involves the patient selecting from a menu of appropriate treatment options presented by the doctor, who has a duty to offer treatments which will benefit the patient. Choice involves both the doctor and patient, working in partnership, weighing the benefits and harms of the various alternative treatment options. There is no coercion and the responsibility for the outcome of the choice is shared between the doctor and patient. Such a model of choice or informed consent involves a high level of trust and excellent communication between the doctor and patient to ensure these conditions of free informed choice without coercion are met.[13] However, a different 'market' model of choice is now prevalent in healthcare.[13] Here choice involves competition, protection of the consumer from harm and a menu of almost unlimited choices.

In the traditional model of informed consent the doctor is obliged only to offer treatment choices which she feels are of potential benefit to the patient. In a consumerist market model the practice would be to offer every choice so that patients may choose treatments which were harmful or which had no potential to create benefit. A market model of choice encourages patients to believe they have a 'right to die' and that they may choose the timing and mode of their own death. This right then extends to involve a doctor in assisting them to commit suicide or to intentionally kill them at their own request.

Thus choice is a step towards competition, to shopping around, which is inconsistent with the collectivism of the NHS ethos. The responsibility for the choice lies entirely with the patient (consumer). In this model the role of the doctor is to provide whatever possible treatment the patient chooses rather than the traditional model where the doctor considers which treatments have a realistic chance of benefitting the patient. Increasingly in the UK, the government is adopting the consumer choice model in the NHS. Hospital trusts compete for patients who are encouraged to compare the different hospitals in league tables which claim to demonstrate which hospitals and consultants are 'best'.

The market model is based on a claim that choice will create a more equal society. However, such a model of choice is inherently unfair since it will always be the articulate, mobile, middle-class patients who access these choices, and the vulnerable elderly, who settle for the nearest treatment centre, who will be disadvantaged.

The economic consequences of providing multiple choices can be considerable. To provide choice is to create spare capacity and hence wasted resources. Quality of care may be threatened in a competitive market as a result of the drive to reduce costs. Moreover, choice is associated with individualism and autonomy whereas equity is associated with collectivism and justice.[14] Therefore choice and equity become competing ethical ideals.[15]

As we have seen, an individual may make a choice for euthanasia or assisted suicide. The attempts to legalise assisted suicide in the UK have sought safeguards to ensure that a choice to die reflects more than a minimal concept of individual autonomy that might reflect momentary desire, lack of comprehension, or a lack of information or even coercion. It is doubtful whether legislation can specify all the criteria that may be important in making such a choice. Legislation has to be framed to protect all citizens, not simply tailored for hard cases while risking the lives of others.[16]

However, in reality, choices cannot be objective; compassion is often and understandably mixed with frustration and even anger and even with hopes and interests in another's death. Thus true informed consent cannot reliably be achieved in this situation. Even deferential and frightened choices are choices, but they are only minimally autonomous and are not fully informed and understood. Patients with advanced cancer may choose aggressive treatments, with unpleasant side-effects, just to pacify their families and to be seen to be fighting the cancer. Choice may be affected by the beliefs of friends and relatives rather than reflecting the autonomous wishes of the patient. The media can drive choice and induce hysteria by depicting dying as necessarily involving pain, suffering and indignity. Such fears can be a strong motive behind a patient's request for assisted suicide. It is interesting that although the patient may choose to have assisted suicide it is the doctor who ultimately decides whether the patient's choice is respected. In the Netherlands 20% of euthanasia requests are turned down by the doctor who judges that the patient is not 'suffering enough'.[17] This surely is a denial of patient autonomy.

The traditional model of choice or informed consent infers a joint responsibility since the doctor takes responsibility for the treatment options and the patient then chooses to consent or refuse. The consumer choice model forces the doctor into supplying treatments which she believes are futile. The doctor is just doing what the patient wants, overriding the doctor's autonomy, and the autonomy of others who might be influenced by the individual's choice. A switch has taken place; it is now the doctor who consents and the patient who authorises. This consumerist model leads to the demise of professionalism, compassion, integrity and altruism. Consumerism has a different ethic from professionalism.

JUSTICE

Justice as an abstract concept is one that is difficult to define with its implicit notions of morality, socially 'correct' behaviour and redress. Justice is a concept which deals with questions about the law, of rules about how individuals should treat each other. Sandel suggests that there are three functions of justice: maximising welfare, respecting freedom and promoting virtue.[18] Sandel argues that moral dilemmas about justice may arise when the three components conflict or when there is uncertainty as to the consequences of an action.[18]

Political philosophy is divided between promoting a virtuous society and allowing people to be free to choose the best way to live. This division reflects the differences between the Ancient Greeks, such as Aristotle, who emphasised virtue, and modern thinkers promoting freedom of individual choice.

In *Antigone* it may seem initially that it is Antigone who is 'right' and Creon who is 'wrong'. However, Antigone might have made a different choice had she known that her choice would result in not only her own death but the suicide of her fiancé and that of his mother.

Antigone is brought to the king, Creon, and in her final words says:

> 'Never I tell you. If I had been the mother of children
> Or if my husband died, exposed and rotting –
> I'd never have taken this ordeal upon myself,
> Never defied our people's will.'

These lines can seem confusing: what does Antigone mean? Is she expressing remorse for her actions at the end? Most critics feel that she is merely emphasising that her conduct was a matter of personal choice. Her duty to her brother was so strong that it overrode any other consideration and took no account of the consequences to others.

In contrast, Creon, widely depicted as the villain of the play, feels that his law protects the welfare of Theban society: 'Whoever places a friend above the good of his own country, he is nothing. . . . Remember this: our country is our safety.'

Thus he justifies his decree that Polyneices' body should be left exposed: 'No, he must be left unburied, his corpse carrion for the birds and dogs to tear, an obscenity for the citizens to behold.'

Moral reasoning about justice is not simply an individual matter but involves a wider public debate.[18] Crucially, this involves us in listening to those who have different views from our own. Odone describes the movement to legalise euthanasia to be largely driven by 'the chattering classes', a middle-class group who have only a superficial understanding of the issues involved and who ignore the potential consequences of a change in the law.[19]

Creon fails to listen when his son Haemon, who is betrothed to Antigone, begs him to reconsider his decision. Haemon tells his father that the people of Thebes are unhappy with his decision to execute Antigone. Creon refuses to take any account of the people's views. The fact that there is a popular call to change the law should be reason for informed moral debate and not by itself sufficient reason to make the change. It is important as doctors that we understand that social and cultural 'norms' are often deeply embedded, and an attempt by an 'outsider' to challenge these tenets can be met with mistrust or antipathy. In a Chapter 9 on *Behzti* we will observe how a young female Sikh playwright has attempted to shed light on coercion and abuse that is apparently happening 'behind closed' doors in a particular cultural environment.

Creon will not be moved even when his son threatens suicide. Later he stubbornly refuses to reconsider his decision when Tiresias, the blind seer, tries to warn him of the errors of his ways. It is only when the Chorus points out that he should listen to wise advice that Creon hastily tries to save Antigone. But Creon is too late, Antigone is hanged and then Haemon kills himself in despair. Creon returns home broken, only to find that his wife Eurydice has also killed herself. The tragedy lies in the loss of meaning; it is the needless ending of lives with potential that is the essential tragedy of *Antigone*.

A MODEL OF AUTONOMY, CHOICE, DIGNITY AND JUSTICE

This analysis of *Antigone* and the clinical story of a patient who requests euthanasia highlight the complex way in which autonomy, choice, dignity and justice interact. Two models of the interaction between these concepts emerge: a narrow 'market' approach and a broader 'responsibility' approach.

The narrow 'market' model

Autonomy is characterised by independence and self-centredness. Choice is entirely self-serving and justice allows the individual complete freedom to choose whatever they judge is best for themselves. Dignity here is seen to be related to a functioning body and independence from others. This model stresses rights rather than responsibilities or duties.

The broad 'responsibility' model

This model accepts that there are limits to respecting individual autonomy, such as a choice which has the potential to harm others. Autonomy is grounded in dependency upon others. Our autonomy is reflected in our relationships with friends, family and the state, and it is this relational aspect which carries the sense of responsibility for our decisions. Autonomy is not striving for self-assertion but is a reflective concept which takes account of the broader narrative of members of the community in which we live.

Choice is related to informed consent, a process whereby the doctor and patient come to a joint decision based on honest information which is

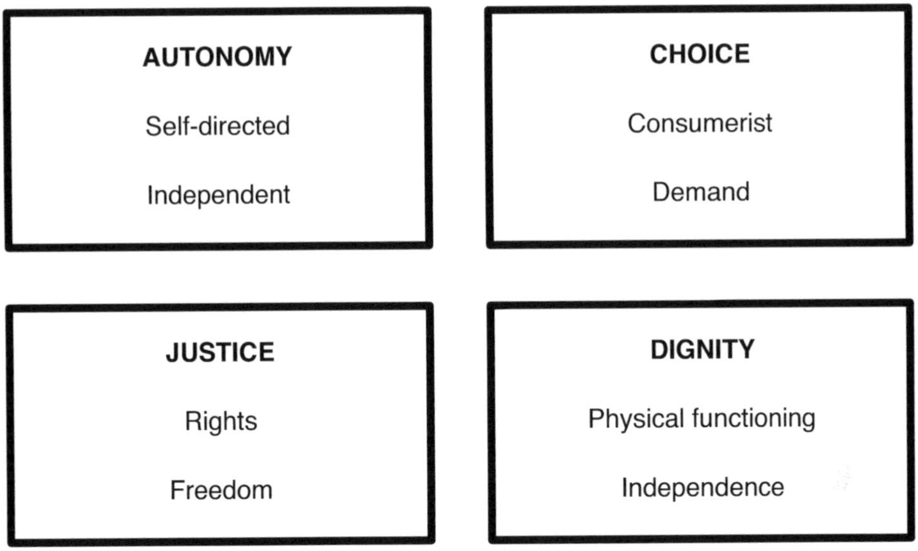

AUTONOMY	CHOICE
Self-directed	Consumerist
Independent	Demand

JUSTICE	DIGNITY
Rights	Physical functioning
Freedom	Independence

FIGURE 4.1 The market model

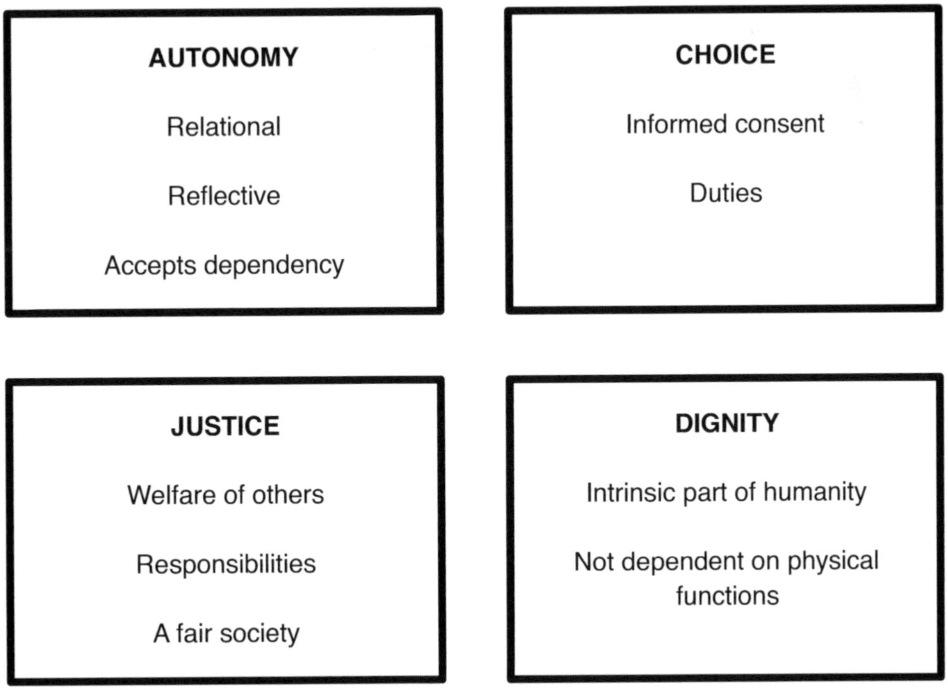

AUTONOMY	CHOICE
Relational	Informed consent
Reflective	Duties
Accepts dependency	

JUSTICE	DIGNITY
Welfare of others	Intrinsic part of humanity
Responsibilities	Not dependent on physical functions
A fair society	

FIGURE 4.2 The 'responsibility' model

understood. Choice is affected by responsibility and duties rather than appealing to rights. Justice takes account of the welfare of others and strives towards the promotion of a fair society.

Dignity is intrinsic and does not depend upon physical characteristics but rather is an integral part of being human.

Our study of *Antigone* explores the moral dilemmas which arise when principles of autonomy, choice, justice and dignity conflict in situations where the consequences of our actions are uncertain. Our models identify why such conflicts may occur and therefore help us to reach wiser decisions in clinical practice. The clinical case of a request for euthanasia was chosen because doctors are faced with continuing to support and care for a patient when they cannot agree to their choice for a hastened death. The many different moral and practical arguments involved in the debate about the legalisation of assisted suicide and euthanasia are beyond the scope of this book but are discussed elsewhere.[20,21]

CONCLUSION

People in Western societies are privileged to have unprecedented levels of choice about almost every aspect of their lives. While they can influence their health through their lifestyle choices they still have little choice in the timing, place or manner of their dying.[22,23] We have looked at issues surrounding a choice of the timing of one's death, and it is not surprising that many of the reasons for wanting that choice arise in the context of choice of place of death.

It is ironic that although most people wish to die in their own home, only around 20% of patients with cancer in the UK achieve this wish, despite a rise in the provision of community palliative care over the past 30 years.[22]

General practitioners are offered incentives to record their palliative patients and to raise the issue of their preferred place of death. This can be difficult for some doctors who may fear upsetting patients and so avoid these discussions. Other challenges are that for a choice to be realistic the patient should have a range of alternatives: home, hospital, nursing home or hospice. In reality these may simply not be practical. The other problem is the difficulty in predicting when death will happen, particularly in non-cancer diagnoses such as heart failure or advanced lung disease. The picture becomes more complex since a patient's choice can change with time.[22] Factors influencing a change in choice include social support, perception of being a burden to carers, fear of loss of dignity and the views of their carers.[23] Just as in choices surrounding a hastened death, there was uncertainty about what the future might hold for them. Each person has their own individual expectation of the dying process and this seems to be an important factor in determining their choices. Furthermore, while some patients are content to discuss their choices about dying others remain in denial and many others will be ambivalent.[24] Discussions about this choice may only achieve a preference towards 'home' or 'hospital' rather than a definitive answer.[25] Munday points out that the tick-box approach that GPs are required to fill in a form as part of their palliative care Quality Outcomes Framework risks ignoring the ambivalent changing nature of a patient's choice by simply recording 'wishes to die at home'.[22]

In the examples we have studied of choices in end-of-life care, either in the place of death or the timing of death it is clear that in ordinary medical practice patients' choices are limited by both what is medically deemed appropriate, by organisational issues and by time.[26] Patients cannot choose any treatment they wish; they only have a formal right to refuse treatment. Some of the complexity within the concept of autonomous choice is that what may be perceived as a single decision often involves many different people over a period of time. This makes it difficult to identify who has the moral responsibility for the decisions. Often patients do have a choice, but it is within a narrow framework set by the doctor in advance.[26] Thus the presence of choice in itself does not mean the patient is being respected or empowered. Processes of informed consent designed originally to protect patients from paternalistic doctors in medical research do not necessarily easily transfer into clinical practice. In the latter situation patients are sick and are dependent on assistance and choices may have to be made when time for reflection is limited.[26] Perhaps our model of responsibility gives autonomy an important place but does not restrict autonomy to the presence of choice but draws a wider framework to mean respect for the person. A responsibility model serves to bridge the potential gap between medical practice and medical ethics which the choice-dominated consumerist model creates.

REFERENCES

1 Higgins C. Harridans, harlots and heroines: women of the classical world. *The Guardian.* Available online at: www.guardian.co.uk/lifeandstyle/2010/oct/08/harridans-harlots-heroines-women-classical (accessed 16 January 2013).

2 Brennan C. On the road to howling ruin. *The Guardian.* Available online at: www.guardian.co.uk/stage/2008/oct/26/antigone-manchester (accessed 16 January 2013).

3 Ince WN. Prologue and Chorus in Anouilh's *Antigone. Forum for Modern Language Studies.* 1968; **IV**(3): 277–84.

4 Watt L. *Attic and Elizabethan Tragedy.* London: JM Dent & Sons; 1908.

5 Gillon R. *Philosophical Medical Ethics.* London: John Wiley; 1985.

6 Dworkin G. *The Theory and Practice of Autonomy.* Cambridge: Cambridge University Press; 1988.

7 Kant I. Groundwork of the metaphysic of morals. In: Paton HJ, editor. *The Moral Law.* London: Hutchinson's; 1948.

8 Keown J. *Euthanasia, Ethics & Public Policy.* Cambridge: Cambridge University Press; 2002.

9 Groenewood JH, van der Heide A *et al.* Clinical problems with the performance of euthanasia and physician assisted suicide in the Netherlands. *N Engl J Med.* 2000; **342**: 551–6.

10 Taylor C. *The Ethics of Authenticity.* Cambridge, Massachusetts: Harvard University Press; 1991.

11 Sulmasy DP. Dignity and bioethics: history, theory, and selected applications. In: The President's Council on Bioethics, *Human Dignity and Bioethics: essays commissioned by the President's Council on Bioethics.* Washington, DC: The President's Council on Bioethics; 2008. Available online at: www.bioethics.gov/reports/human_dignity/index.htm

12 Chochinov HM. Dignity and the essence of medicine: the ABC and D of dignity conserving care. *BMJ.* 2007; **335**: 184–7.

13 Downie R, Randall F. Choice and responsibility in the NHS. *Clin Med.* 2008; **8**: 182–5.

14 Barr DA, Fenton L, Blare D. The claim for patient choice and equity. *J Med Ethics.* 2008; **34**: 271–4.

15 Oliver A, Evan JG. The paradox of promoting choice in a collectivist system. *J Med Ethics.* 2005; **31**: 187.

16 O'Neill O. *Autonomy and Assisted Suicide Living and Dying Well.* (17 August 2010) Available online at: www.livinganddyingwelll.org

17 Haverkate I, Onwuteaka-Phillipsen BD *et al.* Refused and granted requests for euthanasia and assisted suicide in the Netherlands: interview study with structured questionnaire. *BMJ.* 2000; **321**: 865–6.

18 Sandel M. *Justice: what's the right thing to do?* London: Penguin Books; 2010.

19 Odone C. *Assisted Suicide: how the chattering classes have got it wrong.* Centre for Policy Studies; 2010.

20 Warnock M, Macdonald D. *Easeful Death.* Oxford: Oxford University Press; 2008.

21 Jeffrey D. *Against Physician Assisted Suicide: a palliative care perspective*. Oxford: Radcliffe Publishing; 2008.

22 Munday D, Dale J, Murray S. Choice and place of death: individual preferences, uncertainty and the availability of care. *J R Soc Med*. 2007; **100**: 211–15.

23 Higginson I, Sen-Gupta GJA. Place of care in advanced cancer: a qualitative systematic literature review of patient preferences. *J Palliat Med*. 2000; **3**: 287–300.

24 Townsend J, Frank A, Fermont D *et al*. Terminal care and the patient's preference for place of death: a prospective study. *BMJ*. 1990; **301**: 415–17.

25 Thomas C, Morris S, Clark D. Place of death: preferences among cancer patients and their carers. *Soc Sci Med*. 2004; **58**: 2431–44.

26 Agledahl KM, Forde R, Wifstad A. Choice is not the issue. The misrepresentation of healthcare in bioethical discourse. *J Med Ethics*. 2011; **37**: 212–15.

CHAPTER 5

Change: *Little Eyolf*, Henrik Ibsen (1894)

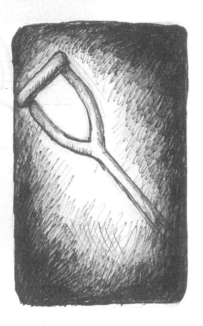

Norwegian playwright Henrik Ibsen's masterful study of guilt and bereavement, *Little Eyolf* (1894) explores the tensions and recriminations between Alfred and Rita, a married couple whose disabled son drowns. Ibsen's drama is known as 'Symbolist', whereby visual metaphor is used to drive the narrative: later in this chapter we will look at these particular metaphors. While Ibsen's drama was often controversial at the time of writing, his psychological exploration of desire, guilt and blame are still acutely relevant today and have constructive applications to end-of-life care. The critic Michael Billington states: '[The play] was the product of a lifetime's obsession with the idea that spiritual regeneration could be achieved by confronting the darkest truths about oneself.'[1]

SYNOPSIS

Alfred Allmer has been visiting the mountains in order to clear his head and consider his plans for his young son Eyolf, who has a limp. He has decided to try to encourage Eyolf to pursue an intellectual path, as his disability will prevent him from engaging in physical pursuits. The play opens with Rita and Alfred's sister Asta discussing Alfred's holiday and Eyolf's struggles. Alfred and Eyolf enter. Alfred seems in good spirits as he tells Rita that he has spent his time thinking rather than working on a book he is writing. Eyolf talks about his wish to travel to the mountains and discusses the physical activity he wants to take up. We learn that Eyolf plans to be a soldier when he is older. Ominously, Asta announces that she has seen the Rat Wife, a drifter who claims to be able to drive rats away from houses. The characters discuss the myths surrounding the Rat Wife. Alfred tries to encourage Eyolf to go to the beach to play with the other boys, but Eyolf refuses, claiming the boys will make fun of his smart clothes.

Silently, the Rat Wife enters, asking the family if there are any 'gnawing things' that are troubling them. At Alfred's invitation, the Rat Wife sits and rests as she tells the family rather ghoulishly about the 'jobs' she has done freeing houses from vermin. She shows Eyolf the little dog she keeps in her bag to help lure the rats out to the sea to drown. Eyolf is fascinated by the dog, and the Rat Wife hints that having been jilted by her lover, she lured the man to his death. The Rat Wife leaves, and Eyolf follows her, unnoticed. Alfred and Asta discuss the family letters that Asta has been keeping in her portfolio. Alfred asks her about the letters from Asta's mother; Asta tells him that he should keep these as he has not yet read them. There is an uneasy moment, which is compounded when Rita remarks on the 'graveyard' atmosphere that the Rat Wife brought with her.

Rita claims that both she and Asta have noticed that Alfred has changed since being in the mountains. Alfred reveals that he has experienced something of an epiphany by being away from his study and thinking rather than writing his book (which we learn is called *Human Responsibility*). He tells Rita that he wants to be a better father to Eyolf, and to help him to grow emotionally and intellectually. Rita is somewhat taken aback by Alfred's fervour.

The road engineer Borgheim enters, who is romantically interested in Asta. He announces that he has been given a new contract to build a large road across the country, and is in high spirits. He asks Asta if she would like to take a walk with him. Asta initially is reluctant but is pressured by Rita to leave with Borgheim. Before he and Asta leave, Borgheim asks where Eyolf is, and is told he is 'out playing'.

After Asta and Borgheim leave to walk in the garden, Rita and Alfred discuss the possibility that Asta and Borgheim are in a romantic relationship. Rita reveals that she hopes Borgheim will take Asta away with him, as she craves the attention of Alfred alone. Rita becomes very passionate and claims that she believes their son has prevented them from enjoying a happy marriage. Rita goes on to denigrate Eyolf further by claiming he is only 'half' hers. She pointedly reminds Alfred of how she dressed up for him and prepared champagne for his return, but that Alfred did not touch the champagne. Pointedly, she tells Alfred that if he stopped loving her, she would run into the arms of the nearest man; Alfred disagrees with her. Rita is again angered when Alfred mentions Eyolf tenderly, and begins to tell her husband, we infer, that she wishes Eyolf were dead.

Borgheim and Asta return, showing signs of 'restrained emotion'. Borgheim starts to discuss the 'evil eye' with Rita. Rita again makes a derogatory reference to Eyolf, much to Alfred's dismay. The conversation is halted when the group hear shouts from boys outside by the shore of the fjord. It appears a child has drowned; at first the group believe it cannot be Eyolf, but they overhear the phrase 'the crutch is floating' and realise that their son has indeed drowned.

Act 2 begins in secluded countryside next to the fjord. We find Alfred sitting by himself, lost in thought. Asta approaches him and chides him for sitting out in the gloomy weather. Alfred is clearly traumatised, and upsets Asta by talking about the 'depths' of the fjord, and calculating how many hours it has been since Eyolf drowned. Alfred tells Asta that the boys saw Eyolf being lured to his death by the Rat Wife. Asta tries to soothe Alfred and sews black crepe onto his hat. We learn from Asta that Borgheim has come to town, as he was fond of Eyolf. The pair reminisce and Alfred reveals that if Asta had been a boy she would also have been called Eyolf, and they fondly recall their childhood when Asta would dress up in boys' clothes and Alfred would call her 'Eyolf'. Alfred then expresses guilt that he has forgotten momentarily about the death of his own son, but Asta reassures him and says that Eyolf has influenced his memories. Asta is shocked when Alfred says he wants to go down to the fjord and prevents him from going. They discuss their family life, and Alfred expresses his admiration for Asta and we glean that they have always been very close as siblings. They turn their conversation towards the parents, and it appears that their father was distant and cruel to their mother. Asta asks Alfred to go to Rita, but Alfred clearly draws solace from Asta and clasps her hand, calling her his 'big Eyolf'.

Rita and Borgheim arrive. After trying unsuccessfully to get Alfred to accompany them, Asta takes Borgheim away to leave the grieving couple in peace. Rita tells Alfred that she is haunted by the image of her dead son, lying deep in the clear water with wide open eyes. She did not see him herself, but is relying on the memories of the boys who saw Eyolf drown. Alfred and Rita begin to argue, with Alfred asking his wife if Eyolf's eyes were 'evil'. Alfred remonstrates with Rita, claiming that she wished Eyolf dead, which Rita denies. Rita claims that Asta had damaged her relationship with her son, as Asta always took Eyolf to her heart. She then accuses Alfred of never having loved Eyolf, and being obsessed with the writing of his book. Alfred rounds on Rita, and claims that it is she who made Eyolf disabled, and therefore unable to save himself from the water (we understand later that Eyolf acquired his disability when he fell off the table while his parents were making love).

The argument becomes more impassioned when Alfred reveals that he dreamed of Eyolf running without any disability, and he wanted to offer thanks. Rita asks him whom he would thank and we understand Alfred is an atheist, and Rita bitterly comments that his atheism has taken away her own faith and thus a source of comfort in their grieving. Alfred asks Rita if he were to take his own life and was guaranteed to be with Eyolf would she do the same. Rita denies that she would, and Alfred agrees that their place is with the world of the living. Rita suggests 'forgetting' the pain and anguish that Eyolf's death has caused or holding loud parties so their senses will be dulled. Alfred rejects these plans and hints that he might take up his writing again, angering Rita further. Alfred tells Rita that Eyolf's dead staring eyes will be constantly watching their relationship, before proposing that there may be some transformative power in Eyolf's death that might bind them closer together. Rita spurns Alfred's argument again, claiming that she does not want 'resurrection'. They turn their focus to the early stages of their relationship, and Alfred confesses that Asta brought them together. Rita reminds Alfred that he told her he used to call Asta 'Little Eyolf': when he confessed this to her, they made love and left their son unattended, causing him to fall from the table and cripple himself. Alfred begins to break down at this memory.

Asta and Borgheim re-enter the scene, Asta holding waterlilies. The arguing couple attempt to preserve a façade of normality. Alfred requests that he speak with Asta alone, Rita agrees and leaves with Borgheim. Alfred then announces to Asta that he can no longer bear to live with Rita. He expresses his desire to live with Asta as brother and sister again, to replicate their childhood. Asta is shocked and unsettled and tells Alfred that he should read the letters from their mother. Alfred begins to ask more questions, and pressurises Asta into revealing that she is not in fact Alfred's sister. Alfred is shocked, but maintains that their relationship is still sacred. Asta gives Alfred the waterlilies, which she has picked from the depths of the fjord, as a last greeting from 'Eyolf'. When Alfred asks which Eyolf (as Asta was also known by this name) she replies that they are from 'both of us'. The act closes with Alfred and Asta returning to the house, with Alfred moaning 'Eyolf'.

Act 3 is set in the Allmers' garden, where there is a bare flagpole. Asta is found sitting on a bench. Borgheim, carrying a rolled-up flag, enters and asks what Asta is doing. She tells him she is taking a last look at the fjord before she leaves. Borgheim says he is hoisting the flag to half-mast at the request of the grieving couple who are apparently spending time apart. He also informs Asta that he is leaving to begin his road building, and that he grieves deeply for Eyolf. Asta reassures him that once he has moved far away his grief will lessen. They decide that they will travel separately, effectively suggesting the end of any romantic relationship. Borgheim encourages Asta to talk about her childhood with Alfred, unaware that the pair are not in fact related. Asta talks warmly of her past with Alfred, before becoming tense when she talks about Alfred marrying, and we have the impression that she felt, or still feels, a sense of abandonment. She tells Borgheim that Alfred has been subject to the 'law of change', which Borgheim dismisses bluntly. Borgheim in turn comments on the 'one blow' that has changed Asta's relationship with her brother. Asta assumes momentarily that this is the news that she is not his sister, but quickly understands that Borgheim means the death of Eyolf.

Borgheim next tries to convince Asta to come with him to help with his road building. Asta asks him if he would be content only to have 'half of her' (implying that she still shares an intimate bond with her 'brother'). Borgheim replies in the negative, and goes to leave. At this point Alfred comes into the garden, looking for Rita. Alfred and Borgheim talk about the flag, before Borgheim announces that he is leaving. Alfred assumes that he will be travelling with Asta, but Borgheim denies this. Alfred remarks on how terrible it is to be alone, and that Borgheim may meet a partner on his travels. Asta tells Alfred that she is going to leave for town and that she will not be coming back to visit in the immediate future.

Rita arrives, and appeals to Borgheim and Asta not to leave. Rita claims to have seen the image of Eyolf's dead eyes staring at her. Alfred begs Asta to stay with them. Rita, too, seems afraid of being left alone with Alfred and her grief. Rita suggests that Asta could fill the void left by their son by becoming their 'little Eyolf'. Asta is upset and impulsively states that she will leave with Borgheim on the steamer, much to Borgheim's joy. She embraces Rita and leaves with Borgheim.

Alfred and Rita are left alone. Alfred asks Rita to look at the departing steamer, but Rita sees the lights as Eyolf's staring eyes. Rita is outraged the steamer is leaving from the same spot where Eyolf drowned. Alfred talks of the 'pitiless' nature of life, and that life goes on, regardless of tragedy. He goes on to talk about how Eyolf has vanished from their world. When Rita tells him the crutch remained, Alfred becomes angry and agitated and tells his wife never to talk about the crutch again. Rita becomes animated and claims she can hear the 'knell' of a tolling bell, and the phrase 'the crutch is floating' rings in her ears. This distresses Alfred further, but he appears to be sympathetic to his wife, claiming that the 'law of change' has affected them, and that they might transcend to a higher life or understanding. Rita suggests Alfred could take up his writing again, something that to this point she has expressed her contempt for. Alfred then proposes that they should break up and he should return to the mountains to live in solitude. He tells Rita that when he was in the mountains, he 'lost' himself and found that both Rita and Eyolf 'drifted' from his thoughts;

he also embraced the 'luxury of death'. Rita finds his story upsetting, more so when Alfred describes death as his 'fellow traveller' who came to take Eyolf away.

Rita expresses her concern that Alfred will leave her, but they are interrupted by 'quarrelling' noises. Rita believes they may have found Eyolf's body, but Alfred rejects this, claiming he will never be found. The noise turns out to be fighting on the shore, and Rita proposes that Alfred intervenes. Alfred becomes bitter, remarking that the same boys fighting were the boys who did not help Eyolf. He asserts that he must now be harsh for Eyolf's sake. Yet Rita feels the opposite, and says that she wants to take the boys in and look after them. They both agree that as a couple they have not been socially responsible. Alfred agrees to Rita's plan, and they state their belief that this will stop Eyolf's death being in vain. Alfred tells Rita that her plan is not borne out of love: Rita agrees and says it is to appease Eyolf's piercing eyes. The play ends in a moment of intimacy and tenderness as the couple stare up to the night sky and the 'great silence' as Rita gives her husband her hand and thanks him.

MODERN INTERPRETATIONS AND CULTURAL CONTEXTS

Little Eyolf was reinterpreted by playwright Samuel Adamson as *Mrs Affleck* in 2009. Adamson transplanted the action to the Kentish coast in 1955 and anglicised the characters. This reinvention did not appear to excite the reviewers. The critic David Benedict's remarks are typical of the general response to the play:

> Despite Adamson's breadth of compassion, the actors' energies cannot stop Mrs Affleck from feeling besieged, largely because both the old and new texts have too few events to keep their ideas moving forward. Less adherence to Ibsen's plotting might have allowed Adamson's new interpretation to take wing.[2]

Billington also was critical, and asked 'Why not simply re-stage *Little Eyolf*?'[1]

We live in a society where patterns of mourning and the 'right behaviour' are often held up to scrutiny by others. In *Behzti* we observe how Min is trapped within a rigid socio-religious system that relies on notions of 'honour', with dissent being met with brutal reprisals. *Cloud 9* also represents fixed social structures that are reinforced by prejudice and assumption: the young Edward, being male, is remonstrated for wishing to play with dolls; Kathy is herself reduced to the status of a doll as her autonomy and opinions are denied to her. In *Journey's End* the soldiers must mask their fear of death by talking about mundane subjects: showing their natural fear would be stigmatised.

Yet, conversely, we can observe how society is mistrustful of those who do not show their emotions in the wake of trauma and bereavement. In 2007, the disappearance of Madeleine McCann shed light on a disturbing propensity for society to cast judgement on the 'correct' way to grieve. Madeleine's parents were frequently the target of newspaper articles that insinuated that because the couple appeared to be outwardly calm and collected, they must therefore have had a hand in their daughter's abduction or murder. This kind of rhetoric was also apparent in the 2001 case of Peter Falconio who vanished while travelling with his girlfriend Joanne Lees in the Australian outback. Suspicions were raised by Lees's apparently relaxed demeanour: surely someone recently bereaved must display deep distress?

It might be useful here to return to Pinter's remark that 'the more acute the experience, the less articulate the expression'. In *Little Eyolf* we see how both Rita and Alfred are tortured by their inability to communicate their personal grief at the loss of their son and find themselves hobbled by social expectation and compromised by the tenets of religious faith. Somehow, however – as in *Blasted* – by the end of the play the couple find a form of transcendence and resilience in the same vein as the character in Samuel Beckett's novel *The Unnameable* who says, 'You must go on, I can't go on, I'll go on.'[3]

CHANGE

In the Introduction we referred to Aristotle's notion of *peripeteia* or 'change' as a central catalyst for the plot of a drama, embodied in this instance by the enigmatic and eerie Rat Wife who will lure Eyolf to his death. It is possible that the Rat Wife herself represents death entering the Allmers' household, as Rita remarks: 'Ugh! I feel as if that horrible old woman had brought a sort of graveyard smell with her.' Clearly, Ibsen is reinventing the traditional Pied Piper figure (who also abducted children) yet the Rat Wife also serves to highlight the Allmers' embedded marital tension and guilt about Eyolf's disability when she asks if they 'are troubled by any gnawing things in the house'. The arrival of a stranger and consequent disruption of order is repeatedly seen in Pinter's work: consider Davies' intrusion in *The Caretaker*, or the arrival of the sinister henchmen Goldberg and McCann in *The Birthday Party* who arrive to remove the surrogate 'son' Stanley. Goldberg ominously remarks that 'if we didn't come today, we would have come tomorrow'. This sense of inevitability infuses Ibsen's play where symbols of death (and also renewal) are repeatedly employed: from the posie of waterlilies that Asta gives to Alfred, to Rita's imagining of the Eyolf's 'evil eye' staring up from the bottom of the fjord.

The play explores how the characters cope with, or resist, change. Alfred's abortive book is tellingly entitled *Human Responsibility* and we are shown how both he and Rita struggle with taking responsibility for Eyolf's welfare as well as in a sense accepting responsibility for his death. But the play also investigates the dimensions of social and technological change through the character of Borgheim who is contracted to build a major new road to link the cities across Norway. It is Borgheim who manages to form a connection with Asta and their departure for a new life together, reinforcing the possibility of renewal, or a 'fresh start'.

It is clear that the 'change' that affects Rita and Alfred is psychologically devastating and leads to reprisals. What is also evident is the 'management' of bereavement: the couple are careful to shield Asta and Borgheim from their expressions of pain and as such their mourning is apparently carefully controlled.

CLINICAL PERSPECTIVES

In this chapter we explore the changes associated with bereavement, in particular the loss of a child. The emotional responses related to loss are described as grief, while mourning describes the process of adaptation to bereavement.[4] If we love others, inevitably we will experience the pain of grief when they die. Since palliative care is centred on both patients and their families, bereavement support forms a core part of this care. Although most grieving is painful it can be a time of personal growth, despite the sadness of the loss. However, there are situations where bereavement can result in abnormal or complicated grief reactions. Insights gained from *Little Eyolf* can help healthcare professionals to support bereaved families and hopefully to prevent complicated grief reactions by recognising risk factors for abnormal grieving patterns and providing appropriate extra support. Various models of bereavement have been devised to try to give healthcare professionals a theoretical structure to make some sense of the grieving process and to help them to devise appropriate interventions to support the family. To complicate the picture of grieving, culture may also influence grieving with different emotions, rituals and expectations of privacy or public mourning.

It is beyond the scope of this book to detail all the bereavement models but the salient features of some of the more pragmatic models are outlined in this chapter. Attachment theory suggests that parental bonding generates a sense of security in the child. In *Little Eyolf* the bonding between Eyolf and his parents is weak. Alfred feels guilty that he has neglected his son and resolves to be a better father by spending time with him rather than writing his book.

'I cannot divide myself in this matter – and therefore I efface myself. Eyolf shall be the complete man of our race. And it shall be my new life-work to make him the complete man'.

Rita admits: 'Then I wish he had never been born.'

Bowlby's attachment theory proposed that the nature of the bonding influences the impact of the loss.[5] In *Little Eyolf* both parents feel guilty about their emotional distancing from their son so are at risk of complicated grieving when confronted by the traumatic loss.

Interpersonal theories focus on the ambivalence felt towards the deceased and suggest distress is heightened when these feelings predominate.[4] In *Little Eyolf* Rita is jealous of Alfred's attention and concern for Eyolf. Rita threatens to throw herself into the arms of the first man who comes her way:

> RITA: For then I should take him away from someone else; and that is just what Eyolf has done to me.
> ALFRED: Can you say that our little Eyolf has done that?
> RITA: There, you see! You see! The moment you mention Eyolf's name, you grow tender and your voice quivers! Oh, you almost tempt me to wish–

Rita does not say the words but is silently expressing her anger and wishing her son were dead. Almost immediately after this exchange we learn of the poignant discovery of Eyolf's crutch and that he has drowned.

Later in Act 2 Rita accuses Alfred of not having loved Eyolf:

> RITA: That is just it! I cannot endure to share anything with anyone! Not in love.
>
> ALFRED: We two should have shared him between us in love.
>
> RITA: We? Oh, the truth is you have never had any real love for him either.

Rita castigates her husband for being absorbed in his book, ironically titled *Human Responsibility*. Alfred then admits that there is an unspoken issue between them.

> ALFRED: There is something you shrink from saying.
>
> RITA: And you too.
>
> ALFRED: If it is as you say, then we two have never really possessed our own child.

The 'elephant in the room' is the guilt they both feel as a result of Eyolf's accident when he fell off the table as they were making love.

The couple hear that a child has drowned:

> ALFRED: It isn't Eyolf! It isn't Eyolf, Rita!
>
> RITA: Hush! Be quiet! Let me hear what they are saying!
>
> (Rita rushes back with a piercing scream, into the room.)
>
> ALFRED: What did they say?
>
> RITA: They said: 'The crutch is floating!'
>
> ALFRED: No! No! No!

This captures the disbelief and shock at first hearing the news of Eyolf's drowning.

In Act 2 Alfred cannot come to terms with the fact Eyolf has died: 'No, I cannot grasp it. It seems so utterly impossible.' At first he fears he is going mad, a parallel here with *King Lear*: 'Is it really true Asta? Or have I gone mad? Or am I dreaming? Oh, if only it were a dream! Just think, if I were to waken now!'

The bereaved search for some sense of meaning. Alfred says: 'For, after all, there must be a meaning in it. Life, existence – destiny, cannot be so utterly meaningless.'

Later Alfred expresses his anger at the Rat Wife who he blames for luring Eyolf to his death: 'Why should she? There is no retribution behind it all – no atonement, I mean. Eyolf never did her any harm. He never called names after her; he never threw stones at her dog . . . the whole thing is utterly groundless and meaningless . . !'

It is this meaningless suffering that is hardest to bear.

Sociological bereavement models look at the choice between moving on to new relationships or maintaining an attitude of 'the broken heart'. These models build on the loneliness of grief and emphasise the importance of family and friends in reaching an acceptance and moving on.[4]

In the closing scene of *Little Eyolf* Rita tells her husband that she is going to look after 'the poor neglected children' who live locally. Albert is at first shocked – 'In our little Eyolf's place' – but then reflects how little they have done for the poor people in the past. Rita and Albert conclude that if they can do something to help these children, 'Eyolf was not born in vain' and, as Rita says, 'nor taken from us in vain'. Bereaved parents may find that one way of coping with their loss is to invest time and energy in helping others; often involving themselves in charities associated with the condition their child died from or helping a local children's hospice.

Traumatic grief such as Eyolf's sudden death often results in the intrusion of distressing images and thoughts into the memories of the bereaved. Rita imagines she hears the words 'The crutch is – floating. The crutch is – floating'. She appeals to Alfred: 'Oh, surely you must hear it, too!' but he hears nothing. Rita is haunted by the memory of Eyolf's staring eyes under the water. 'I want to make my peace with the great, open eyes, you see.'

Bereavement models try to make sense of chronic grief where people become stuck in their distress and cannot move on. Stroebe and Schut proposed a model which described the emotional tensions in mourning.[7] They suggest that during the process of coping with loss, the bereaved person moves between two emotional states: loss and restoration. In one state, loss, there is focus on the loss itself with all the distress and suffering this involves. In the other state, restoration, the focus is getting on with life and moving forwards. Stroebe and Schut maintain that the active confrontation with loss is in a dynamic equilibrium with avoidance of grieving in the restoration phase. One of the practical consequences of their model is that people need time out from their grieving.

CLINICAL CASE

Jim and Sally's youngest daughter Naomi died in her cot at six months of age six weeks ago and no cause was found for her sudden death. Sally searches for photographs of Naomi to fill her overwhelming sense of loss. However, when she finds the photographs she is distraught with grief and puts them away, promising herself that she will not look at them again and gets on with her work as a primary school teacher. For a while it seems as if Sally is coping well by immersing herself in work, but Jim finds her at home searching the attic for a suitcase containing Naomi's baby clothes. 'I just have to try and find her again,' Sally explains, breaking down in tears.

In *Little Eyolf*, Alfred feels guilty for forgetting Eyolf for an instant:

ALFRED: He slipped out of my memory – out of my thoughts. I did not see him for a moment as we sat talking. I utterly forgot him all that time.

ASTA: But surely you must take some rest in your sorrow.

For some bereaved parents the pain is so great that they have an urge to join the dead child.

ALFRED: All my thoughts must be out there, where he lies drifting in the depths.

ASTA (following him and holding him back): Alfred – Alfred! Don't go to the fjord.

ALFRED: I must go out to him! Let me go Asta! I will take the boat.

ASTA (in terror): Don't go to the fjord, I say!

ALFRED: No, no – I will not. Only let me alone.

Normal grieving is a form of suffering with physical, psychological and social components. Emotional distress is episodic and involves crying, ruminations about the deceased and the whole spectrum of moods from anger, guilt, fear, anxiety and despair. Alfred describes his 'crushing, gnawing sorrow'.

Asta points out that 'Time will make it all seem easier, Alfred'.

And Alfred responds by asking, 'But how am I to get over these terrible first days?'

Later Rita says 'that horrible sight that will haunt me all my life long. Yes, with great, open eyes. I see them! I see them now!'

Alfred then confronts Rita:

> ALFRED: Now things have come about – just as you wished Rita.
> RITA: I! What did I wish?
> ALFRED: That Eyolf were not here.
> RITA: Never for a moment have I wished that! That Eyolf should not stand between us – that was what I wished.

Alfred admits: 'Sorrow makes us wicked and hateful.'

As they argue the parents accuse each other of not loving Eyolf. Rita observes: 'Yes, isn't it curious that we should grieve like this over a little stranger boy?'

They then blame each other for the fall when Eyolf was a baby which resulted in the damage to his leg. In their grief neither is able to support the other.

> ALFRED: It was you that left the helpless child unwatched upon the table.
> RITA: And you had promised to look after him.
> ALFRED: And now, what we now call sorrow and heartache – is really the gnawing of conscience, Rita. Nothing else.
> RITA: I feel as if all this must end in despair – in madness for both of us. For we can never –never make it good again.

The bereaved may feel a sense of outrage that the world seems to carry on as if nothing had happened. As they watch the boat moor by the pier where Eyolf drowned, Alfred says, 'Life goes its own way – just as if nothing in the world had happened.'

Personal loss is often difficult to reconcile with an apparently indifferent world. The conflict between private suffering and a broader sense of life carrying on has fascinated writers and artists over the years, from Brueghel's painting *The Fall of Icarus* where the drowned man appears as a small detail in a wider rural landscape to Chekhov's *The Seagull* where a suicide is presented almost as a footnote to the narrative.

One important practical consequence for healthcare professionals helping to support the bereaved is to remember to acknowledge the loss and not to suggest that the dead child will be forgotten and the parents will get over it. Alfred and Rita consider separating but later decide to stay together and help the poor children who live locally.

Physical expressions of grief may include numbness, restlessness, loss of appetite, sleeplessness, weight loss and loss of energy. The bereaved may behave in ways reflecting the loss–restoration model: socially withdrawing, then searching and seeking the dead person, finding reminders, experiencing pain and to repeat the cycle by retreating into isolation again.

Grieving can be abnormal, a syndrome classified as complicated grief, characterised by intense separation distress and persistent protest against the death. Also, to meet diagnostic criteria for this syndrome, four of the following possible symptoms must be experienced daily and persist for at least six months: non-acceptance of the death, feeling life is meaningless, lack of trust, anger, pessimism and inability to carry out daily activities.[4]

In palliative care bereavement support is particularly targeted at those at risk of complicated grief. Risk factors of complicated grief, which alert healthcare professionals, can be identified in *Little Eyolf*. Complicated grief is associated with highly dependent and ambivalent relationships, such as that between Eyolf and his parents. This is a result partly of his disability and also his parents' guilt. Both Rita and Alfred have ambivalent feelings about their son, another predisposing factor for abnormal grieving. Eyolf's sudden, unexpected and traumatic death and the fact that it occurs in an untimely fashion, before that of his parents, make complicated grief more likely.

Alfred and Rita have a dysfunctional relationship. Rita says: '. . . you will leave me – for you think it's only here, with me, that you have nothing to live for'.

Bereaved people who feel alienated and isolated are more likely to have prolonged complicated grief reactions than those with strong networks of family support. The unspoken guilt about Eyolf's fall indicates that communication between Rita and Alfred is not open and honest but closed and distancing. One of the most difficult aspects of parental bereavement is that the death of the child hits both partners simultaneously and confronts them with overwhelming loss.[6] Instead of being there to support each other, each partner is working through their own grief. Some parents may try to replace a dead child and experience survivor guilt.[4] Rita and Alfred plan to help the local poor children at the end of the play.

Although the death of a child is not something to 'get over', grieving can be followed eventually by a process of adaptation which can be accompanied by personal growth. The death of a child creates an empty space for the surviving family.[6] Rita and Alfred talk of 'an empty place within them' and they feel a need 'to fill it up with something that is a little like love'.

However, the bereaved can emerge from mourning with a renewed sense of meaning, increased empathy and new goals and values.

MODELS OF GRIEVING AND TASKS OF MOURNING

Stroebe and Schut's Dual Process Model[7] may be combined with Worden's Practical Tasks of Mourning[8] to give a helpful framework for healthcare professionals to understand the grieving process. Stroebe and Schut illustrate grieving as a dynamic process in which the tasks described by Worden are accomplished in a fluctuating manner, not a linear progression, through stages in any defined order. This model also suggests that bereaved people need space for a break from their grieving as they oscillate between the two phases of loss and restoration.

CONCLUSION

As we have observed in Chapter 3, doctors need to be able to connect and share the distress of those they are attempting to help. This connection is a way of showing compassion. Yet when confronted by the emotional distress of caring for a dying child, professionals sometimes distance themselves by 'doing' behaviours in an effort to maintain self-control. With experience and support professionals gradually discover what they can do to alleviate suffering. By working in an interdisciplinary supporting team doctors can build their confidence in their ability to remain connected and care for dying children and their families without disengaging.[6] Perhaps the most important lesson for healthcare professionals helping bereaved parents is that they cannot take away their pain and suffering. Instead they must value 'the gift of presence', of being there, to share suffering.[6]

Writing in *The Washington Post* in the aftermath of the shooting of the school-children in Newtown, Connecticut, Ann Hood reflects on the needs of grieving

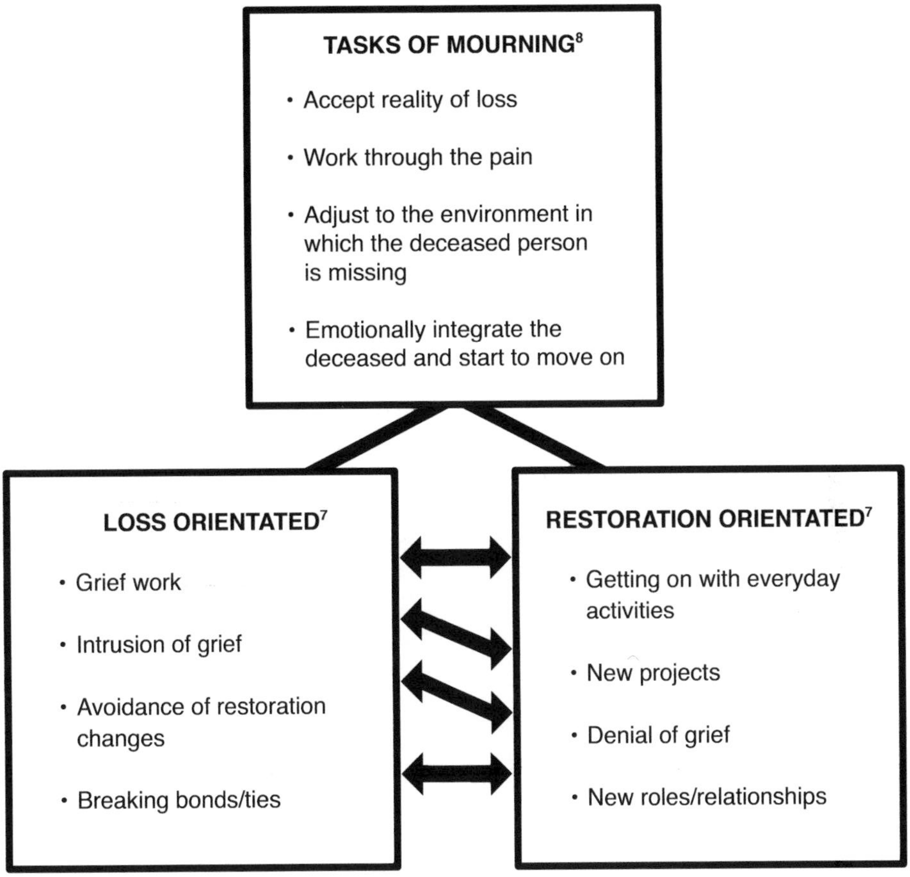

TASKS OF MOURNING[8]

- Accept reality of loss

- Work through the pain

- Adjust to the environment in which the deceased person is missing

- Emotionally integrate the deceased and start to move on

LOSS ORIENTATED[7]

- Grief work

- Intrusion of grief

- Avoidance of restoration changes

- Breaking bonds/ties

RESTORATION ORIENTATED[7]

- Getting on with everyday activities

- New projects

- Denial of grief

- New roles/relationships

FIGURE 5.1 Models of grieving

parents, those left behind.[9] She writes about 'an enormous hole that is left forever' and reflects that no one can give the parents what they want most – their child. As a bereaved parent she writes: 'I have learned there is more power in a good strong hug than in a thousand meaningful words.'[9] Friends who just sat and listened to her talk, wail and curse were particularly appreciated as were those who remembered and used her deceased daughter's name. She acknowledges that the grief of the parents of the children killed in this shocking tragedy will never completely go; it will always be there. She gives advice to others seeking to comfort and support them: 'Do not forget that. Look them in the eye. Take them in your arms and do not let them go.'[9]

REFERENCES

1 Billington M. Mrs Afflick, Cottesloe, London. *The Guardian*. Available online at: www.guardian.co.uk/culture/2009/jan/28/mrs-affleck-cottesloe-review-ibsen (accessed 16 January 2013).

2 Benedict D. Available online at: www.variety.com/review/VE1117939500/?refCatId=1265 (accessed 16 January 2013).

3 Beckett S. *The Unnamable*. New York: Grove Press; 1958.

4 Kissane DW, Zaider T. Bereavement. In: Hanks G, Cherny N, Christakis N *et al.*, editors. *Oxford Textbook of Palliative Medicine*. 4th ed. Oxford: Oxford University Press; 2010.

5 Bowlby J. The making and breaking of affectional bonds. *Br J Psychiatry*. 1977; **130**: 201–10.

6 Davies B, Orloff S. Bereavement issues and staff support. In: Hanks G, Cherny N, Christakis N *et al.*, editors. *Oxford Textbook of Palliative Medicine*. 4th ed. Oxford: Oxford University Press; 2010.

7 Stroebe M, Schut H. The dual process model of coping with bereavement; rationale and description. *Death Stud*. 1999; **23**: 197–224.

8 Worden W. *Grief Counselling and Grief Therapy: a handbook for the mental health practitioner*. New York: Springer; 1982.

9 Hood A. Death of a child: a parent's worst nightmare. *Washington Post*. Available online at: http://articles.washingtonpost.com/2012-12-21/opinions/36017342_1_worst-nightmare-gun-control-grief (accessed 15 January 2013).

CHAPTER 6

Concealment: *All My Sons,* Arthur Miller (1947)

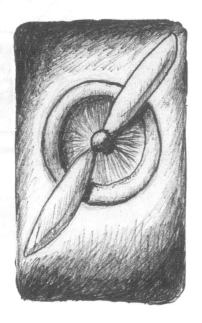

MOTHER: Joe, you're doing the same thing again; all your life whenever there's trouble you yell at me and you think that settles it.

All My Sons

INTRODUCTION

All My Sons is one of the most significant plays not only in Arthur Miller's canon but in the context of American theatre in the landscape of drama in the 20th century. An uncompromising deconstruction of both greed and the capitalist dream, the play charts one man's guilt-ridden descent into a personal hell where he must accept that his actions have had fatal consequences. Joe Keller is outwardly a gruff but kind paterfamilias, yet harbours a dark secret under the veneer of social respectability. For Joe's factory has been producing faulty aircraft parts which has resulted in the death of 21 pilots. Joe himself has escaped reprisals while his business partner still languishes in jail for the crime.

Miller's plays often share particular themes such as a buried past that returns to haunt a character, the pressures of society to conform, the failure of the American Dream to protect the individual and the hidden tensions within the nuclear family. In this chapter we will explore *All My Sons* with a particular emphasis on the notion of concealment, and more specifically how a failure to disclose information or feelings may result in the denigration of the individual. We will draw clear parallels between the dynamics of Miller's play and the tensions which can arise when giving patients information concerning their diagnosis, treatment options or prognosis.

This is another play in our chronology where family bereavement (and denial or acceptance of loss) is in the foreground. Much of the tension within the play is generated by the degree to which the characters accept that a young family member is dead. The mother, Kate, is adamant throughout the play that her son Larry (a pilot) is alive, despite being missing for three years. The other characters are placed in difficult psychological situations as they try to negotiate with her, without hurting her feelings. As well as focusing on the central character of Joe Keller, we would like to explore this form of silent communication (and concealment) in some detail and relate these dynamics to end-of-life care. We will also explore, in both the play and the palliative care context, how personal feelings of 'guilt' can be damaging both to the patient and their family.

PLOT SYNOPSIS

The three-act play is set solely in the back yard of the Kellers' house; we are informed that this is in the outskirts of an American town. Joe Keller, the patriarch and notional head of the household, is reading the paper with his friend Jim Bayliss. We learn that a tree, planted in memory of their pilot son Larry who is missing in action in the Second World War, has blown down in a storm. The atmosphere is initially fairly jovial. The neighbour Frank appears to tells Joe he is going to try to work out Larry's horoscope for the day he went missing, to see if it is a 'favourable day'. We are introduced to Frank's wife Lydia, as well as another neighbour, a nurse called Sue. Joe is characterised as warm-hearted as we watch him play a 'cops and robbers' game with Bert, a small boy from the neighbourhood.

Chris, Joe's son, enters and tells Joe he has invited Ann (Larry's ex-girlfriend) to the house in order to ask her to marry him. Joe expresses concerns, firstly that Chris's mother will strongly disapprove (Kate refuses to believe Larry is dead and therefore he is still in a relationship with Ann); he then is dismayed that, once married, Chris intends to leave the Keller family business. Kate enters and appears distressed at the felling of Larry's tree; she also insists that Ann believes Larry is still alive and remains faithful to him, despite Chris's protests. She also appears disproportionately angry that Joe pretends playfully that there is a jail in the house, to amuse Bert.

Ann arrives. Kate again maintains that she is still in a relationship with Larry. We learn that Ann's father, Steve, is in jail, and that he was in business with Joe. Joe, rather complacently, talks about the court case that saw him exonerated and welcomed back into society while Steve was (and is still) incarcerated. The case surrounded the manufacture, by Joe's factory, of cracked cylinder heads for P40 aircraft. It appears that Steve had sanctioned the sale of these defective parts without Joe's knowledge, resulting in the death of 21 pilots. Ann asks Joe if he is angry at Steve for 'dragging him through the mud'. Joe appears breezy and forgiving about Steve's behaviour. Ann raises the possibility that Larry was killed as a result of her father's crime, which causes Kate to become even more distressed. Joe staunchly defends Steve and claims the man is not a 'murderer'. Ann and Chris are left alone on stage. Chris professes his love for Ann and the couple embrace and agree to marry, Ann ready to move on from her memories of her relationship with Chris's brother. Joe returns and gently mocks the couple for their amorous behaviour. Chris tells Joe that he and Ann intend to marry. Act 1 ends on an ominous note as Ann receives a phone call from her brother George who is a lawyer and has visited their father in jail. George is keen to visit the Kellers and tells Ann that he is taking the next flight from New York. Joe appears unsettled and awkward as the act closes.

Act 2 begins with Kate in a troubled state, believing Ann's family to have antipathy towards her own. Chris attempts to reassure her. They go into the house together; Ann enters and is met by neighbour Sue who is strangely belligerent. She tells Ann that she hates living next door to the Kellers because of their success, and that Joe, while admired for his business acumen, is seen as morally bankrupt. Ann and Chris return, and are again interrupted by Joe who tells Ann that he'd like to offer Steve a job at his factory when Steve is released. Jim enters to warn Chris that George is coming to take Ann away from the family, but he is cryptic about the reasons. George finally arrives and tells the family that he has spoken with his incarcerated father, and that his father told him that it was Joe who ordered him to cover up the cracked cylinder heads, and that Joe wouldn't come and resolve the situation as he was 'in bed with flu'. The tension is lifted slightly when Kate enters and is kind towards George, but George continues to press his point and challenge Kate with the claim that Joe was never ill with flu at that time. Frank appears and tells Kate that he has finished studying Larry's horoscope and that it was a favourable day for him. Overjoyed, Kate packs Ann's bag and asks her to take it and leave. She reasserts to Chris that Larry is alive, because if he is dead it means his father (Joe) must have killed him with his disastrous cover-up of the faulty parts.

Joe, under pressure, finally confesses to an outraged Chris that he did indeed sanction the sale of the faulty parts, but claims he didn't believe they'd ever be used in the planes. When pressed further he asserts that it was a business decision only, and that he did it for Chris's future financial security. The act closes with a short, furious monologue from Chris where he condemns his father as 'worse than an animal' for his actions.

The short, final third act represents a devastating coda to the preceding action.

The act begins with Kate waiting for Chris to return home, and talking with Jim. Jim leaves as Joe enters the yard. Joe states that he doesn't like Jim getting involved in their family matters, but Kate tells him that Jim already knows the truth about the aircraft parts. Kate asks Joe to tell Chris that he is willing to go to prison for his actions. Joe claims this wouldn't solve anything, and again emphasises his positive financial contribution to the family, and that Larry would understand his business-mindedness if he was still with them.

Jim leaves, and Ann returns. She tells Kate that she knows for a fact that Larry is dead because she has his suicide note, which she shows Kate, who becomes very distressed. Chris returns and tells Kate and Ann that he is going to leave permanently as he always suspected that the house and business his father built was based on his father's deception over the aircraft parts.

Joe comes from the house and tells Chris that he should just give his money to charity, and reaffirms that going to jail wouldn't help the situation, and in fact would damage the livelihoods of many other businesses. Chris, exasperated, reads Larry's suicide note to Joe, in which Larry squarely blames Joe for the deaths of his fellow soldiers. Joe, a broken man, goes into the house. Kate asks Chris what purpose sending his father to jail would serve now the war is long over. At this point a shot is heard inside the house as Joe takes his own life. The play ends with a distraught Chris being comforted by his mother.

MODERN INTERPRETATIONS

All My Sons is a harrowing play, and unconventional in its apparently truncated final act that offers us no form of resolution.

Robinson writes: '[The] troubling, abrupt ending fails to resolve the problems the play has posed; and we are left with a survivor incapable of asserting the authority required to restore the symbolic connection with other men he has broken.'[1]

Yet this sudden, dispiriting ending is a natural result of the series of denials that have plagued the family. Kate's central refusal to admit Larry is dead creates a series of related tensions: Chris's relationship with Ann is made furtive and illicit as romance between the two would confirm Larry's demise; more disturbingly, Kate remarks to her son:

> 'Your brother's alive, darling, because if he's dead, your father killed him. Do you understand me now? As long as you live, that boy is alive. God does not let a son be killed by his father. Now you see, don't you? Now you see.'

Joe Keller is also in denial. He abrogates his personal responsibility for the manufacture of the faulty aircraft parts ostensibly to prioritise the commercial benefit from the process, and financial gain for Chris. Many characters invoke money as a justification for jettisoning ideals and hopes; the doctor and Keller both use this justification. One of the many ironies in *All My Sons* is that though Larry was not killed directly by a cracked cylinder head, Joe is still responsible for his son's death, having driven him to suicide.

Jim Bayliss, the family friend of the Kellers, astutely summarises the key dynamic of deception at work in the family:

> JIM: Don't be afraid, Kate, I've always known.
>
> MOTHER: How?
>
> JIM: It occurred to me a long time ago.
>
> MOTHER: I've always had the feeling that in the back of his head, Chris . . . almost knew. I didn't think it would be such a shock.
>
> JIM (gets up): Chris would never know how to live with a thing like that. It takes a certain talent . . . for lying. You have it, and I do. But not him.

Jim is hinting here that there may be situations where it is morally permissible to lie. We will explore this idea later in this chapter.

CLINICAL CONTEXT

People depend upon honest information in order to make decisions. We trust a stranger to be honest if we stop to ask directions. It is perhaps ironic that doctors, who are trusted members of society, may be viewed with some suspicion by their patients when it comes to being truthful. Historically, doctors could act paternalistically and lie to patients, for example in concealing their true diagnosis, by claiming 'therapeutic privilege'.[2] This privilege was used when doctors felt that the patient would be harmed if they were aware of the seriousness of their condition. A doctor would avoid using the word 'cancer' or might not disclose a poor prognosis. However, over the past 40 years it has become accepted in medical ethics that the patient has a 'right to the truth'. With the increasing emphasis on patient autonomy has come a realisation that one important way of respecting such autonomy is to give honest information. Furthermore, the concept of informed consent relies on the fact that the patient gives permission for a medical intervention on the basis of honest information which they have received and understood.

Novak has shown that there has been a huge change in doctors' behaviour with regard to telling patients the truth. In 1961, he found 90% of doctors did not reveal a fatal diagnosis to patients, but by 1977 97% of doctors were honest about informing the patient about such a diagnosis.[3] A more recent study of resident physicians' attitudes about the use of deception revealed that the majority (90%) would disclose the truth, in this case about medical errors.[4]

Patients need to know their diagnosis, the proposed treatment, together with the risks and potential benefits of any proposed intervention. They also should be made aware of the alternative treatments possible and the potential consequences of their refusal of the suggested treatment. There are a number of ways in which this process may be threatened.

The first difficulty for the doctor is to know what is meant by the 'truth'. In some cases of diagnosis this might be clear, such as when breaking bad news about the diagnosis of leukaemia from a blood sample. However, as we have seen in previous chapters, much of medicine relies on probabilities and is uncertain. So while it may be relatively simple to be truthful about the diagnosis it is much more uncertain when discussing the prognosis with an individual patient. The doctor faces the difficulty in communicating this uncertainty without being obstructive and failing to meet the patient's wish to know what is going to happen to her.

Doctors may react into the question 'How long have I got?' in a number of ways.

They may just say, 'I cannot be sure, no one knows.' This is an example of a truthful response but one which does little to help the patient.

Alternatively, they may explore the patient's beliefs and reasons why they need to know. The patient with leukaemia may say, 'I had a grandmother who had leukaemia and she lived for 10 years with her disease . . . will that be how it is for me?' Or, 'I want to see my children into school next term. Will I live until then?'

By avoiding assumptions and trying to understand the patient's view the doctor comes to understand how to best communicate uncertainty and to respond as honestly as possible so that the patient can make realistic choices. Truth telling, whether about a life-threatening diagnosis or a poor prognosis involves the emotions of the doctor and the patient as well as relatives who might wish to protect their family member from the harsh reality.

It is not simply the content of the message which is relevant ethically but the manner in which it is given. A doctor might be 'brutally honest' and deliver a life-threatening diagnosis in a sudden way to an unprepared patient who will then react with shock and denial. In this situation the patient has not come to terms with the reality of their situation and the doctor has failed to communicate effectively. In practical terms this behaviour has resulted in concealment of the diagnosis from the patient's point of view.

A patient may see their GP after being in hospital and although the doctor has a letter to say the patient is aware of their diagnosis, the patient looks up blandly and says, 'They did not tell me what was wrong.' This common situation exemplifies the complex emotional aspects surrounding truth telling.

Some research on patients with lung cancer shows that doctors and patients may enter a collusion to talk only about the treatment plan rather than discuss the reality that the cancer will eventually recur and kill them.[5] This collusion occurs not because the doctors have not tried to be honest but rather that the patient has not allowed them to pursue this line of honest discussion.

Typically in the outpatient clinic, after results show recurrence of cancer despite the chemotherapy, the patient looks up at her oncologist and asks, with a hopeful smile, 'OK so this last treatment has not been successful, so what's next doctor?'

The doctor may feel that ethically it would be a neglect of their duty not to harm the patient by removing all hope so he might respond: 'Well, we could try some further experimental treatment. I can't promise it will work but . . .'

'Thank you doctor, you know I am a fighter. Let's go for it.'

The doctor has effectively concealed the poor prognosis and is now committed to prescribing futile chemotherapy as a way of maintaining hope.

Another way of lying which doctors may use might be labelled as being 'economical with the truth'. The use of medical jargon or false optimism might be examples of how this can be done:

- 'The patch on your chest X-ray has not resolved completely. We need to give another course of chemotherapy to clear it up.'
- 'It is so difficult to say how long you have got; it's a bit like how long is a piece of string?'
- 'The operation on your bowel cancer was a success. I am pleased to say we got it all removed.'

In many clinical situations the doctor is torn between honestly informing the patient so that informed autonomous decisions can be made and protecting them from the 'harm' of hearing bad news. Ethically, the doctor has to decide between the principles of autonomy and beneficence. If he decides that the information would cause unnecessary suffering he can give the latter a priority and claim a 'therapeutic privilege' to lie to the patient. If a doctor is going to lie to a patient he could justify this ethically by appealing to a Utilitarian calculation and claiming that he was maximising happiness by withholding the truth. On the other hand, a Kantian approach would regard lying as inherently immoral and thus the doctor would have to apply the strict standards of informed consent and always give honest information.

Sokol suggests a practical way forward to reconcile formal ethical considerations and the emotional realities of clinical care.[6] The first step is to identify that the information shared with the patient conceals the known facts. The next step involves a reflection of the reasons why the doctor chose to conceal the facts. Is the concealment likely to increase the patient's well-being or prevent significant suffering? Lying can only ever be justified if it is for the patient's good. It is never justified to conceal information simply because breaking bad news causes the doctor discomfort. Valid reasons which could possibly justify concealing information might include a wish to give the patient time to come to terms with their situation, by presenting chunks of information at a time rather than giving all the facts at once. Other situations in which concealment might be justified are when the patient is highly anxious, depressed or feeling hopeless. In considering how to act the doctor must pause and reflect on the true reason for concealment and ensure that he is not withholding the truth because he lacks the communication skills to deliver the information in a sensitive manner which the patient could accept. The default position is to tell the truth because concealing the truth denies the patient of her right to know and overrides her autonomy. Furthermore, the doctor must consider other results of lying which might be that the patient will make a poor decision based on inadequate information and may be angry and feel betrayed when they discover the truth later. In the study by The *et al.*, mentioned earlier in this chapter, many patients felt angry when they eventually discovered that the treatment they had received had been futile.[5]

Another important consideration in debating truth telling is the effect of lying on the patient's trust. If the doctor is discovered or even thought to be lying, the patient may lose trust and become even more anxious. 'This is so scary that even the doctor is frightened to discuss it.'

The next step for the doctor to consider is what the patient's view would be on concealment or lying. Although over 95% of patients expect and want the doctor to give them truthful information, there remains a tiny minority who do not want all the facts and seem happy to leave medical decision making to the doctor.[7] It can never be assumed that the patient is one of this tiny group and the doctor must continue to check at different times to see whether the individual patient does want more information. Asking the family about truth telling is usually unhelpful as they naturally want to protect their relative from further distress and will often say, 'The news would kill her. She's not good at being ill. Please don't tell her how serious it is.' If the doctor goes along with this request a situation of collusion is created which results in the patient becoming even more isolated emotionally from their family and carers. A final test of a doctor's justification for lying might be to reflect on whether they would be happy to defend themselves in the event of a complaint.

It is perhaps counterintuitive but some patients find it difficult to adjust if they are given bad news about a fatal cancer which turns out to be incorrect and they do not have a life-threatening disease. 'You need to prepare to die,' a patient was told in May 2010.[8] This presents the patient with a confrontation with the limits of their own mortality, sometimes called 'existential angst'. However, in this case, the patient did not have terminal pancreatic cancer and when he was told the 'good news' he 'felt numb'. 'I just couldn't get my head round the transition from focusing on dying to living.'[8] Subsequently, he became depressed and only after a year began to appreciate life again. This example raises ethical issues surrounding survivorhood. In a study of 15 patients Pascal looked at the ethical challenges of a cancer diagnosis. He found the uncertainty surrounding diagnosis, investigation and subsequent treatment served as a 'wake-up call' and precipitated ethical challenges.[9] Among these, patients were faced with finding meaning in survivorhood. Some patients found that quite apart from diagnostic outcome, tests themselves have the capacity to create fear and stress and highlight their fragile position.[9]

However, other patients found this process sometimes was beneficial, in that there seemed to be positive aspects to the experience of having cancer as well as the obvious negative ones. As Pascal comments, 'It is in the everyday world, going to work, reading, cooking and gardening that patients feel the most impact of their cancer diagnosis.' Patients 'are pulled out of the soothing rhythms of life into an angst-inducing and ethically rocky terrain'.[9]

Survivors questioned the purpose of their lives, often asking moral questions about living a good life. This rethinking is not easy but is a key feature of the existential challenge of survivorhood.[9] The consequences for survivors were that they learned the limits of their boundaries with others and this increased connection with others through self-acceptance: 'This is the way I am'.[9] Compassion for others was increased through the patients' experience of their own suffering. Patients need opportunities to tell their story and in doing so to find meaning.

GUILT AND JUSTICE

Guilt in *All My Sons* is realised in a number of different ways which may resonate with patients, their family and the medical team. Further, in our Chapter 4 on *Antigone*, we explored the notion of justice and its relationship to the society in which it is embedded.

In Miller's play, Joe has apparently escaped a form of conventional legal justice by allowing his colleague to take full criminal responsibility for his actions. For doctors, the issue of professional competence can be a threat. Joe's crime is one of negligence, which he attempts to justify in the closing stages of the play by claiming that he never believed the faulty parts would be used. His acceptance of guilt is poignant when he acknowledges that he had a paternal and professional responsibility for the welfare of Larry's fellow pilots: 'Sure, he was my son. But I think to him they were all my sons. And I guess they were, I guess they were.'

We may infer from this that Joe's acceptance is more than legal culpability; it is an acceptance of his responsibility as a human being to a wider society.

It may be useful to draw a parallel here with JB Priestley's socially progressive play *An Inspector Calls*, where an otherworldly detective interrogates a complacent affluent family over the suicide of an impoverished young woman, Eva, in whose death they have all been complicit. The inspector's final lines to the family echo Joe's realisation of his social responsibility:

'One Eva Smith has gone – but there are millions and millions and millions of Eva Smiths and John Smiths still left with us, with their lives, their hopes and fears, their suffering and chance of happiness, all intertwined with our lives, and what we think and say and do.'[10]

In Priestley's play, no character has evaded justice in a legal sense: their 'crimes' manifest themselves in callousness and a lack of social compassion.

Justice involves fostering attitudes and virtues, such as honesty, on which a good society depends.

CONCEALMENT AND SILENCE

Concealment is rife in *All My Sons*. We talked in the introduction of Aristotle's dramatic notion of *peripetaia*, meaning 'reversal of fortune' or 'discovery'. Clearly, the most significant concealment to be 'discovered' is Joe's knowledge of his own guilt about the faulty aircraft parts. But there is a form of complicity in this concealment from the 'team' that surrounds him. After all, Jim confesses that he has 'always known' about Joe's guilt. Like JB Priestley's socially progressive play *An Inspector Calls* (where each member of an apparently 'happy', affluent family has a key secret that is disclosed as the play progresses), Miller sets up the family environment initially as one that is seemingly idyllic and relaxed, and through the course of the narrative exposes the hidden tensions that lie beneath. As we have seen in previous chapters, silence is effectively deployed in an attempt to expiate these tensions, but it is precisely this silence that generates even more distress as the characters are psychologically torn apart by a sense of guilt.

In Chapter 5 we looked at guilt and silence in Ibsen's *Little Eyolf* where a couple try to suppress their feelings of responsibility and anger. Alfred Bates writes: 'We may detect in Ibsen a certain cynical satisfaction in discovering the worm in the apple, the flaw in the diamond, the rift in the lute.'[11]

While we may not call Miller 'cynical' as his plays demonstrate a deep compassion for his flawed characters, the playwright takes care to expose the characters' secrets at a measured pace, allowing the audience to understand the cause and effect of guilty silence.

With the exception of Chris, no character attempts to challenge Kate over her claim that Larry is still alive. This is arguably because this silence will pre-serve the status quo, and allow the mother to indulge her fantasy. But, as we have seen, Kate overtly states that she cannot accept the truth of the situation, because that would have unbearable implications: that is, that Joe was respon-sible for their son's death.

Joe, too, is silent about his guilt for the majority of the play, and instead tries, somewhat pathetically, to emphasise his compassion and kindness by insisting that he will offer his jailed partner a job in his firm.

In the previous chapter on *The Caretaker* we explored the notion of silence and inability to act. In one of Pinter's earlier plays, *The Birthday Party*, the hapless, swaggering lodger Stanley is subjugated and abducted by the sinister figures of Goldberg and McCann. The playwright states: 'All Stanley had to do was to admit to himself who he was. If he had done so, Goldberg and McCann would never have come. Or if they did, the outcome would be very different.'[12]

Shakespeare's famous line from *The Merchant of Venice* – 'the truth will out' – is pertinent both to the dramatic worlds of Ibsen, Pinter and Miller, but also to a clinical context. The more the characters attempt to suppress the truth, the more they are undermined and disempowered. But there will come a point where there is disclosure – this forced disclosure is more damaging due to the previous systematic suppression of the truth.

What we witness in *All My Sons* is the attempt to avoid speaking the truth in order to prevent a disruption in the day-to-day running of the family. But this silence is insidious, because it creates tensions and divisions as there is osten-sibly 'nothing to talk about'. Chris feels guilty about his new happiness a form of survivor guilt.

CASE HISTORY

In palliative care it is common for relatives to try to persuade doctors to conceal a life-threatening diagnosis or short prognosis from the patient.

Jim is dying with lung cancer and the doctor thinks that he has only a few weeks to live. Before he goes in to see Jim on a home visit, he is stopped at the foot of the stairs by Betty, Jim's wife, who says, 'Please don't tell him how bad things are, Doctor. He would just give up.'

This places the doctor in a difficult position. His duty is to be honest with

Jim yet he also has to support Betty in her caring of her husband. He takes time to sit down and explore why Betty wants to conceal the truth from her husband. He also establishes how hard it is for Betty and the rest of their family and friends to keep up this pretence. The uncomfortable silences and lies drive a wedge in their relationship at a time when they most want to be close and loving. The doctor acknowledges that Betty is concealing the truth because she loves Jim and wants to protect him from the harsh reality. However, Betty needs to consider two other factors. First, that Jim probably has a good idea that he has not much time left to live and is probably trying to protect her by putting on a brave face. Second, if he does not realise yet he will probably be very angry when he finds that he has been deceived.

The doctor also says that he has always had a good trusting relationship with Jim and this is threatened if Jim perceives that his doctor is not being honest with him. The doctor explains: 'I am not good at lying; Jim will know that I am being evasive.'

The doctor suggests to Betty, 'Look, if he asks me about the future I will ask him what he thinks and if it turns out that he has a good idea of his situation I will confirm it and we can then drop this pretence.'

Betty agrees to this plan but then asks, 'What if he doesn't have any idea of how serious it is?'

The doctor replies, 'In that case I will ask him what he would like to know and I will not rush into telling him the whole picture but take time to give him the information he requests in amounts that he can take in and understand.'

Betty agrees that this is the best way forward and when the doctor speaks to Jim it becomes clear that he knows that he has only a short time to live. The couple are grateful to the doctor that he has helped break their silence and given them the opportunity to say goodbye in a good way.

MODEL: HONESTY IS THE BEST POLICY

The ethical issues may be summarised in the following way:

Justifications for lying

- Duty of beneficence (to do good)
- Paternalism (I know what's best for you)

- Therapeutic privilege (the doctor can lie)
- Utilitarian justification (consequences – best for everyone especially the patient)
- Altruism.

Justifications for honesty

- Respect for autonomy (respect for individual)
- Right to know
- Need honest information to make rational choices
- To give informed consent
- Protect against paternalism
- Deontological justification: a doctor's duty is to be truthful; no lying is permitted
- Fosters a trusting relationship.

CONCLUSION

The public, patients and their families expect doctors to be honest. The trusting doctor–patient relationship depends on this honesty. We have looked at areas of practice where it may be difficult for the doctor to be honest. However, the real issue is not confined to questions of honesty but also how the truth is communicated to patients and their families. The manner of informing a patient can show respect for their dignity. In Chapter 9 we explore cultural issues in palliative care, but it is relevant to point out here that in some Eastern cultures individual autonomy is not given pride of place. In such cultures there may be patients who expect to be shielded from the truth and in these cases it might be an infringement of their autonomy for the doctor to force unwanted information onto the patient.[13]

If a doctor is considering concealment of information he must first decide for whose benefit it is. Is it for the patient, the doctor, or to accede to a relative?

Patients do not want to be deceived. A doctor may be justified in concealing some facts because a patient cannot handle all the information at once. Skilled communication is necessary to pace the information giving to match the patient's need for information and to check that the information has been understood. Although patients want information about treatment options, they may be happy to defer decision making to the clinician.[14] Davies points out that there may be dangers in mandatory patient autonomy in healthcare. Patients have a right to autonomously choose to let their doctor make the decision based on their medical expertise if that is what they would prefer.[15] They may still require information for a variety of reasons: as part of the general desire we all share to gain knowledge, to make other decisions unrelated to the treatment proposed, to be prepared emotionally and feeling fully informed as a part of respecting their dignity. In contrast, evasive remarks may make the patient feel that they are not respected as autonomous agents. The process of informing provides an opportunity for patients to explore other concerns with their doctor; it is a personal interaction which lies at the heart of the doctor–patient relationship.

REFERENCES

1 Robinson JA. *All My Sons* and parental authority. In: Miller A. *A Collection of Critical Essays*. New York: Chelsea House Publishing; 2007.

2 Richard C, Lajeunesse Y, Lussier M-T. Therapeutic privilege: between the ethics of lying and the practice of truth. *J Med Ethics*. 2010; **36**: 353–7.

3 Novak DH, Plumer R, Smith RL *et al*. Changes in physicians' attitudes toward telling the cancer patient. *JAMA*. 1979; **241**: 897–900.

4 Everett JP, Walters CA, Stottlemyer DL *et al*. To lie or not to lie: resident physicians' attitudes about the use of deception in clinical practice. *J Med Ethics*. 2011; **37**: 333–8.

5 The A-M, Hak T, Koeter G *et al*. Collusion in the doctor–patient communication about imminent death; an ethnographic study. *BMJ*. 2000; **321**: 1376.

6 Sokol DK Can deceiving patients be morally acceptable? *BMJ*. 2007; **334**: 984–6.

7 Meredith C, Symonds P, Webster L *et al*. Information needs of cancer patients in West Scotland: cross sectional survey. *BMJ*. 1996; **313**: 724.

8 Hilpern K. Doctors told Andy Goode he had end-stage cancer and should prepare to die. *Independent*. 14 August 2012.

9 Pascal J, Endacott R. Ethical and existential challenges associated with a cancer diagnosis. *J Med Ethics*. 2010; **36**: 279–83.

10 Priestley JB. *An Inspector Calls*. Oxford: Pearson; 1993.

11 Bates A. *Drama, its History, Literature and Influence on Civilisation*. Kessinger: Whitefish; 2004.

12 Pinter H. Letter to Peter Wood. *Kenyon Rev*. 1981; **3**(3).

13 Pellegrino ED. Is truth telling to the patient a cultural artefact? *JAMA*. 1992; **268**: 1734–5.

14 Manson N. Why do patients want information if not to take part in decision making? *J Med Ethics.* 2010: **36**: 834–7.

15 Davies M, Elwyn G. Advocating mandatory patient 'autonomy' in healthcare: adverse reactions and side effects. *Health Care Anal.* 2008; **16**: 315–28.

CHAPTER 7

Crises: *Blasted*, Sarah Kane (1995)

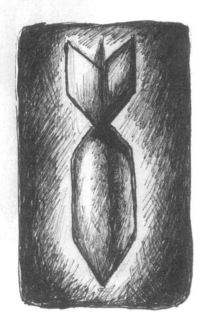

'I'm here, got no choice. But you, you should be telling people.'

Soldier – *Blasted*

In the history of 20th-century theatre, no play has arguably attracted the level of media scrutiny and discussion than Sarah Kane's stark, visceral debut play

Blasted. The graphic scenes of rape and cannibalism combine with an unnerving lyricism (Harold Pinter famously called Kane a 'poet'). Kane took her own life in 1999 after a long history of mental health problems that she explores in her final play, *4.48 Psychosis*.

PLAY SYNOPSIS

Blasted opens in a luxury hotel room in Leeds (the stage directions read that 'the room is so expensive it could be anywhere in the world') and we are introduced to the two protagonists, the foul-mouthed tabloid journalist Ian and his 'partner', the stuttering and nervous Cate (it is clear this is a coercive and abusive relationship). Ian is apparently dying of lung cancer but continues to smoke and drink, peppering his vitriolic and derogatory remarks with casual racism and sexism. Each of the five scenes in the play ends with the sound of rain, and the play ends with a sense of renewal as Ian is fed by Cate. Through the course of the play, we see Ian attempt to rape Cate who manages to escape, before the hotel is hit by a mortar bomb, and the Leeds of the 1990s is transformed into an arena of brutal civil war. This is heralded by the arrival of an armed Soldier who speaks with the same kind of brutality as Ian as he recalls the atrocities that he has committed to civilians during the war, acts of extreme violence, rape and murder. He proceeds to suck out Ian's eyes and rape him before killing himself. Cate then returns with a dead baby she has recovered, and the city is apparently overrun with soldiers. She buries the baby in the floorboards and leaves. The play ends with a series of disturbing images as Ian tries to find some form of comfort, finally eating the baby. Cate then returns and feeds the blinded Ian, who thanks her.

MODERN INTERPRETATION

The play unsettled its original audiences – and indeed the media – not only in its themes, but also the way in which it was constructed. The critic and commentator Aleks Sierz writes: 'if *Blasted* shocked because of its explicit sex and violence, it was also disturbing because of its innovative structure: after a naturalistic first half, Kane exploded theatrical convention by making the second part richly symbolic and eerily nightmarish.'[1]

Sierz further locates Kane's theatre as 'In-Yer-Face', characterised by its 'experiential' style (the audience is confronted with stark reality) and explores themes such as war, intimacy, sexual tension and the role of the media. It is important to note that 'In-Yer-Face' theatre was never a defined 'movement' (the playwrights themselves certainly didn't use this label) but more of general term to look at a series of intersecting concerns from a new generation of writers in a direct but also poetic way.

Kane has stated that the germ of the play was the 1995 massacre of over 8000 Muslim men and boys in the town of Srebrenica in an act of ethnic cleansing. While the play does not specifically reference this atrocity, it is important to locate the play within both the social background and culture of the mid-1990s, while maintaining that the play transcends its Bosnian historical context to offer wider insights into the strength of humanity under unimaginable circumstances.

The play was first performed on 12 January 1996 at the Royal Court Upstairs. Famously, the *Daily Mail* theatre critic Jack Tinker described *Blasted* as a 'disgusting feast of filth', a phrase that rather unfortunately became attached to the piece and surrounding critical discussions. There also seems to be a cultural symmetry between the graphic horror in Kane's debut and the visceral work of the emerging Young British Artists (YBAs) such as Damien Hirst's bisected pregnant calf in formaldehyde, or Marc Quinn's Self – a cast of his head created with pints of his own frozen blood. In an international sense Radovan Karadzic and Ratko Mladic were attempting to hide the scale of their genocide, but a year earlier, in a local context, the grim contents of 25 Cromwell Street and the crimes of serial murderers Fred and Rosemary West were being brought to light.

The historian Hannah Arendt famously coined the phrase the 'banality of evil' in referring to the crimes of the Nazis. It is crucial to note that *Blasted* does not take place in a remote, exotic country but in the mundane surroundings of a British northern city. This apparent incongruity is explored by Harold Pinter in his play *Ashes to Ashes* which focuses on a 'typical' middle-class English couple, where the wife Rebecca appears to have memories of the Holocaust, with her husband, Devlin, becoming her wartime torturer. *Ashes to Ashes* and *Blasted* remind us that brutality and horror are never far away.

It is intriguing to see how Kane has now been absorbed into the canon of Twentieth Century Theatre. There have since been two notable British revivals of the play. In 2001, the play returned to the Royal Court with none of the media 'outrage' that surrounded the premiere. In 2008, the Nineteen Twenty Nine Theatre Company staged the play in a room in The Queen's Hotel, Leeds – apparently Kane's inspiration for the setting – to mixed reviews, with Lyn Gardner in *The Guardian* claiming that 'it is worth remembering that some plays are better served in the theatre'. Kane's play *4.48 Psychosis* has become the *sine qua non* of the Edinburgh Fringe student theatre circuit.

CLINICAL CONTEXT

An initial viewing of *Blasted*, with its uncompromising brutality, might not at first suggest connections with clinical contexts in end-of-life care. It might also be tempting to prioritise Kane's *4.48 Psychosis* (partially informed by her experience of treatment at the Royal Maudsley Hospital) as a more obvious choice in terms of exploring the tensions between dramatic structures and the clinical experience. Yet we would like to propose that there are particular representations of suffering in *Blasted* which can inform and enhance an understanding of the responses of a patient to a crisis. The humiliation of both Cate and Ian raises questions about the nature of dignity. We also highlight parallels with other plays that we have explored in this book.

Arguably, the pivotal moment in Kane's play is when the mortar bomb destroys the haven of the hotel. Prior to this, Ian and Cate have essentially acted in a world that is sealed off from any external reality or responsibility. Ian can indulge in his drinking and bigotry in the comfort of the room, but his sexual abuse of the vulnerable Cate serves to foreshadow the atrocities that the Soldier is later to describe. After the explosion, Ian and Cate's worlds are immersed in complete uncertainty, where the familiar has been reduced to rubble and human survival becomes paramount. Power relationships are changed and new dependencies are created. *Blasted* teaches us about endurance and that in the face of uncertainty, crisis and physical deterioration there can still be hope.

Kane's play is an example of ethical theatre. Morality is aligned with the law and presents us with rules which constrain our behaviour and judges our action and intentions by evaluating them in relation to metaphysical values of good or bad. Ethics, in contrast, is contextual and assesses what we do in relation to particular actions in the particular circumstances we find ourselves in. Ethics encourages us to persevere.

At first sight it may seem that *Blasted* is a depressing play. However, just as we saw King Lear gain insight after enduring crises, so Ian becomes open to possibility following terrible suffering at the hands of the Soldier. He goes through a transformation from an arrogant rapist to a broken dependent man. *Blasted* shows us that good can emerge from the most unfavourable settings and so stimulates us to think about the nature of dignity.

Patients may face crises at various stages of their illness. A life-threatening diagnosis shatters the illusion that we will continue to survive indefinitely. A patient's world may be turned upside down at the time of diagnosis. When the cancer recurs and future active treatment options no longer exist the patient is forced to confront their impending death, the crisis of dying. It is the combination of an unpleasant event with uncertainty in a situation where one feels out of control that can be so stressful.

CRISIS OF DYING

In this chapter we focus on the crisis of dying and to understand this we need to explore what Chochinov describes as the 'landscape of dying'.[2] Physicians need to understand how dying patients may feel if they are to help address their suffering. The crisis of dying raises a number of fears relating to the preservation of dignity, freedom from pain and fears of non-existence. Ian, dying from lung cancer, asks Cate if she is scared of dying. 'You're young. When I was your age . . .' He doesn't finish his recollection, perhaps the fear of dying is too much for him to express. The word 'patient' is derived from the Latin *patiens*, meaning to suffer. The inevitable dependency involved in dying means patients have to surrender some of their autonomy and sense of being in control. They may also experience a loss of their sense of self and so feel a diminution of their humanity: a loss of dignity. They may feel that they are no longer of value and this can cause despair and a sense of hopelessness which contributes to unbearable suffering.

As cancer progresses there may be physical deterioration such as extreme weight loss, limited mobility and changes in appearance. Patients may fear pain which, despite the best efforts of healthcare professionals, may not be completely relieved. The effects of treatment may also cause mutilation, unpleasant symptoms and changes in appearance, all of which can add to a loss of dignity.

In Ian's grotesque blinding by the soldier there is another connection with *King Lear*, just as the play's title may echo Shakespeare's notion of the 'blasted heath'. Douglas Dunn expressed this sense of outrage poetically when he was told that his wife had melanoma in her eye: 'Why there? She's an artist.'[3]

The crisis of dying has psychological, social, spiritual and existential aspects. Although all dying patients experience both sadness and anxiety, psychological responses to a crisis such as a life-threatening diagnosis vary from one individual to another.[4] Therefore treatment approaches must be tailored to each individual patient. Kubler-Ross described, in her classic work, a number of stages or emotional responses to approaching death, with the patient seeming to progress from one stage to another.[5] Initially, there is a period of shock when the person cannot take in the news. The duration of this shock will vary according to the unexpected nature of the crisis and its severity in terms of consequences for the person involved. The period of shock may be followed by a number of differing emotional responses: denial, anger, bargaining, depression and acceptance. Clinical experience suggests that this model is simplistic and in reality people's responses are more complex. Patients may exhibit any of the emotions at any stage and may go back and forth rather than steadily progress towards acceptance. To some extent patients utilise their own coping strategies which they have developed in response to stresses during their life.

In *The Caretaker* we observed how the characters find themselves in a hostile environment, with the 'outside world' being either uncaring or menacing. For Aston, this outer environment has brought only trauma. In Kane's play we see the epitome of the safe 'caring' environment (a luxury hotel) being blown to pieces, leaving the characters prone to assault. In these horrific uncertain surroundings, the characters find themselves having to develop coping strategies in order to survive. What we draw from *Blasted* is the remarkable resilience of the human spirit in the most challenging situations.

Around 25% of all cancer patients will experience severe depressive symptoms, but since diagnosis of depression is often difficult, the condition may be overlooked, so adding to their suffering.[6,7] Although there has been much work on the incidence of formal psychiatric diagnoses such as anxiety and depression in patients nearing death, a sophisticated form of care takes account of more subtle feelings such as hopelessness, feeling a burden to others, a loss of sense of dignity, spiritual or existential angst, loneliness, a desire for death, or a loss of the will to live.[6,8] These feelings may not fit into any psychiatric diagnosis but may cause much suffering. There may also be fears of anticipating pain or a prolonged dying.[9]

In this context it is significant in *Blasted* that the stage directions towards the end of the play read 'Ian dies'. Yet Ian does not die. He endures as a living presence on the stage, and finds a humanity and dignity in thanking Cate as the play closes, indicating a form of transformation or transcendence.

Chochinov observes:

> that within one-to-one interactions with dying patients there are aspects of distress that defy even the most sophisticated of medicinal or technological modalities. Something else is at play and we know it, because it evokes empathy toward our patient's illness experience and resonates with a sense of our common humanity.[10]

Social factors may also be prominent in a crisis. Patients may feel a loss of role and status when they realise that they will no longer be able to work; Ian's loss of sight will mean he will never again work as a journalist. Friends may not keep in touch and then isolation can exacerbate suffering.[11] Changes in one's own body and mood give rise to feelings of loneliness and unfamiliarity toward oneself. In Sand's study when a staff member touched the patient's body in a non-empathic way, this could induce feelings of being treated like an animal.[11] On the other hand, the appropriate use of touch can be a powerful form of 'silent treatment'. Touch can convey empathy, concern and compassion. Care must be taken to respect issues of gender and culture when using touch as a form of silent communication. Touch may also have a therapeutic role in promoting relaxation when used in massage and some complementary therapies.

Kane's visceral play explores the tensions surrounding the body, the self and one's perception of identity. Ian's desires at the start of the play are primal and perhaps 'selfish' (drinking, smoking and ordering sandwiches). Yet he finds himself in a situation where these needs seem insignificant compared with his need simply to survive against a backdrop of assault and terror. In the end, he is fed by Cate, a character whom he has previously dominated and physically abused.

Dying patients may see themselves as a burden to their family and carers and consequently feel that they have less dignity. Caring for a terminally ill person at home can be stressful. Carers need to achieve a balance between caring and coping with their own well-being. Carers can soon feel overwhelmed if they are not supported.[12]

We have seen previously in *The Caretaker* how 'care' is a complex notion, and that apparently 'strong' characters such as Mick also have 'plenty of things to worry about', as well as the pervasive human need for shelter and charity against a world that in itself appears uncaring.

Spiritual or existential crises relate to our universal search for a sense of meaning in our experiences. Patients may ask, 'Why me?' There may be anger directed at their God, at their doctors or even at themselves in an effort to find someone to blame for the crisis. In our secular society both the terms 'spirituality' and 'existentialism' share the human urge to imbue life with purpose, meaning and hope.[13] When a patient is confronted by her own death her priorities change. There is a pause, an opportunity to reflect and to choose to do the things that add the most meaning in the time which is left.[14]

Spiritual pain or existential angst may manifest in subtle ways: denial, unrealistic expectations, demanding futile treatments or requests for a hastened death.[13,15,16] Kissane *et al.* described a 'demoralization syndrome', consisting of hopelessness, loss of meaning, and existential distress. This syndrome can be associated with chronic medical illness, disability, bodily disfigurement, fear of loss of dignity, social isolation and feelings of greater dependency on others or the perception of being a burden to others.[17] Patients can sometimes feel so distressed that they wish for death to relieve them of their suffering.

REQUESTING A HASTENED DEATH

In *Blasted* Ian asks Cate to help him to commit suicide. Ian tries to shoot himself but, unbeknown to him, Cate has removed the bullets from the gun. Cate then claims it was God's will. After the bomb blast we realise what we hope for is impossible; there is a transition from reality to nightmare.

This scene is Ian's 'Dover scene' and corresponds in *King Lear* with Gloucester's request for assisted suicide. A few dying patients do request either euthanasia or assisted suicide to relieve them of their distress.[18] Many of these patients have feelings of hopelessness, are depressed or feel a burden to others. For some it is the fear of future pain or distress rather than any present suffering; these patients have a strong need for internal control.[19,20,21]

Chochinov observes that while palliative medicine has improved the control of pain and other distressing symptoms there remains a need to develop our skills at assessing and engaging with psychosocial, existential and spiritual distress at the end of life.[2] Doctors need to develop an individual approach to each patient, treating them in a holistic manner which means addressing all facets of the illness and life circumstances which may be contributing to suffering.[2] Providing such care presents a challenge since not all suffering can be relieved, even when the best possible care is available. However, suffering may always be reduced by providing time, empathy, presence, compassion and kindness. By giving such care the patient has an opportunity to find meaning, preserve their dignity and address existential or spiritual concerns. With such appropriate care and support some patients find that not all the consequences of having a life-threatening illness are negative. Some describe their terminal phase as being one of the most meaningful times of their lives where they discover new priorities, build relationships and find closure on emotional business.

We all can identify a bad death, but it is difficult to reach a consensus on defining a 'good death' as it varies so much from one individual to another. Chochinov sums up a good death as: 'A meaningful dying process is one during which the patient is physically, psychologically, spiritually, and emotionally supported by his or her family, friends, and caregivers.'[2]

From these observations it seems that care should be directed towards addressing fears of death and dying while respecting and enhancing the patient's dignity or sense of identity as far as possible.[22] Family relationships should be enhanced and conflicts reduced. The patient should be given hope by setting meaningful goals which although limited may foster a sense of continuity with the future. Some patients who request a hastened death may be seeking affirmation that despite their physical deterioration they still are of value. Any notion of suicidal ideation demands that the doctor takes time to sit and listen to the patient, giving them every chance to tell their story and exploring what can be done to relieve their distress.

DIGNITY

Patients facing death often describe a fear of losing dignity, a concept which relates to a sense of self, of one's humanity and connectedness with others.[13] Killminster defines dignity as a capacity for upholding one's principles. She distinguishes two categories of dignity: innate dignity which is a part of humanity and is inviolable, and aspirational dignity which is a state we aspire to and so can be threatened or lost either by our actions or the actions of others or by the situation we are in.[23] Killminster's definition connects loss of dignity with situations of shame or humiliation.

In *Blasted* both Ian and Cate find themselves degraded, the former in his vicious sexual assault by the Soldier, the latter in being forced to use her body simply to get food.

In a medical context this equates with the shame patients feel when their bodies are exposed in wards and in situations of dependency. Although these violations of dignity are not deliberate, they are a source of humiliation.[23] For example, patients are humiliated when they are made to undress in front of doctors, nurses and students. This violation of aspirational dignity results from a surrender of their own standards of public decency which they maintain in their own lives but cannot maintain in an institutional setting.[23]

In *Blasted* torture is used as a way of removing dignity. Ian is both physically and psychologically raped by the Soldier. Ian's rather blasé view of the world in the opening scenes is brutally dismantled by the Soldier's graphic depiction of rape and murder. Under torture people cannot maintain their values; honesty and loyalty are broken. Similarly, in a clinical context, unrelieved pain and loss of bodily functions may compromise the individual's ability to maintain their standards. To be denied the ability to uphold one's personal standards is experienced as humiliation. Killminster argues that we need both concepts: inalienable and aspirational dignity. This has a practical consequence for doctors; it means that they need to be aware that their actions have a profound effect on the patient's dignity and furthermore that their actions have the potential for humiliation. Doctors have dignity too and this also sets limits on their behaviour.

THE CHOCHINOV DIGNITY MODEL

Medical students are familiar with an ABC approach to the resuscitation of the critically ill patient. Chochinov has adapted this acronym to develop a clinical model for enhancing patient dignity: the ABCD of dignity-conserving care.[13] Patients want a human connection with their doctor, and we quote Anatole Broyard again:

> To the typical physician, my illness is a routine incident in his rounds while for me it's the crisis of my life. I would feel better if I had a doctor who at least perceived this incongruity. . . . I just wish he would . . . give me his whole mind just once, be bonded with me for a brief space, survey my soul as well as my flesh, to get at my illness, for each man is ill in his own way.[24]

Chochinov suggests an **ABCD** approach to the distress of dying: A=Attitude, B=Behaviour, C=Compassion and D=Dialogue.[13]

A: Attitude

The attitude of doctors is central to the patient's perception of their dignity. Patients may think they no longer have value and that they have nothing to contribute. This perception of depending on care, while feeling they have little to give back, contributes to a sense of being a burden to others. How patients perceive themselves to be seen by their doctors is a powerful mediator of their dignity.[13] The lesson for doctors is to remember that patients are seeking their affirmation by seeing them as an individual worthy of respect, not just an illness to be managed. Chochinov observes, 'people who are treated like they no longer matter will act and feel like they no longer matter'.[13] As far back as 1927 Francis Peabody wrote: 'One of the essential qualities of the clinician is interest in humanity, for the secret of the care of the patient is in caring for the patient.'[25] Such wisdom reveals that although medical technology has changed a great deal over the past century, human nature remains constant.

Cate's gift is not to abandon Ian, in giving him comfort she allows Ian to live a little longer. Ian is in her debt, but she asks for nothing in return. Cate's presence, touch and compassion, her silent treatments, affirm Ian's value and conserve his dignity despite his mutilation.

Leo Tolstoy wrote about the importance of presence and of honesty in end-of-life care. It may not always be a doctor or nurse who provides this form of silent treatment; it can be a ward clerk, domestic cleaner or tea lady who has time to sit and listen to a dying patient.

> Gerasim was the only one who understood him. It was a comfort when Gerasim sat with him sometimes the whole night through. Gerasim was the only one who did not lie; everything he did showed that he alone understood what was happening, and he saw no need to conceal it . . . and so the relationship was a comfort to him.[25]

B: Behaviour

Once doctors are aware that they play an important role as mediators of patients' dignity, several behaviours should logically follow.[13] Healthcare providers' behaviour towards patients must always be kind and respectful. Small acts of kindness are a way of personalising care and showing the patient that they are valued and respected. Kindness involves connection and is a core part of professionalism; the concept is explored in greater detail in Chapter 3.

C: Compassion

Compassion refers to a deep awareness of the suffering of another coupled with the wish to relieve it.[13] Like empathy, compassion is part of the silent treatment, something that is felt.[13] Compassion may be an intuitive response or may develop with clinical experience. It is a realisation that we are all 'in the same boat', that the patient, like us, is vulnerable in the face of uncertainty. Compassion pervades every chapter of our book and for this reason we have not restricted this most important virtue to a single chapter.

D: Dialogue

Dialogue is a critical element of dignity-conserving care. Communication should acknowledge the individual beyond her illness and recognise the emotional impact that accompanies illness.[13] Listening to concerns and attempting to provide the best forms of care which respects the patient's dignity is a core clinical skill.

CONCLUSIONS

This analysis of Sarah Kane's *Blasted* sheds insight into issues which profoundly affect everyday medical practice. The play examines unbearable suffering, a concept which, in a clinical setting, can only be understood in the context of the patient's perspective of their past, present and hopes for the future. Both Ian and Cate in the play suffer humiliation, which is a violation of their dignity. We have seen that in an extreme crisis patients, like Ian, can request assisted suicide.[27] Medical professionals have a responsibility to deepen their understanding of the individual patient's perspective of suffering, particularly in psychosocial and spiritual domains, so that they can respond to the challenge of this request in an ethical and effective manner. Chochinov's seminal paper describes a model which offers a practical checklist to help professionals respond to patients by respecting their dignity and avoiding humiliation.[13]

Kane has commented on her writing as being perceived as the 'perfect expression of Hell'. The writer Graham Saunders explores the notion of Kane's 'theatre of extremes'.[30] It is in these extremes (extremes of suffering but also of love) that we can understand the complex nature of human dignity and compassion. Owen suggests that the lessons learned by those working in palliative care may have a wider application for people facing any serious crisis in their life.[28] He points to the power of support and helping people to make sense of what is happening. Support also involves help in adjusting to the changes imposed by loss and giving time to allow decisions to be taken. Even in situations of great uncertainty it is possible to make plans which help people regain a sense of control. Finally, and most importantly, healthcare professionals should give emotional support in the face of the storm.[28]

Another psychological approach which can help some patients manage stress and depression is mindfulness meditation.[29] The patient uses their breathing as the focus of attention while observing thoughts, worries and sensations without trying to alter them. Mindfulness is a way of increasing self-awareness, of paying attention to the present moment in a non-judgemental way, of seeing thoughts as thoughts, independently from their content or emotional charge and without trying to replace them with other thoughts or to 'fix' anything.[29] This dissociation of thoughts and feelings from goal-directed action can instil a feeling of freedom.

REFERENCES

1 Aleks Sierz. Sarah Kane. Available online at: www.inyerface-theatre.com/archive7.html (accessed 11 July 2012).

2 Chochinov HM. Dying, dignity, and new horizons in palliative end-of-life care. *CA Cancer J Clin.* 2006; **56**: 84–103. doi: 10.3322/canjclin.56.2.84.

3 Dunn D. *Elegies.* London: Faber & Faber; 2001.

4 Payne DK, Massie MJ. Anxiety in palliative care. In: Chochinov HM, Breitbart W, editors. *Handbook of Psychiatry in Palliative Medicine.* New York: Oxford University Press; 2000. pp. 63–74.

5 Kubler-Ross E. *On Death and Dying.* New York: Simon & Schuster; 1997.

6 Chochinov HM, Breitbart W. *Handbook of Psychiatry in Palliative Medicine.* New York: Oxford University Press; 2000.

7 Chochinov HM, Wilson KG, Enns M *et al.* Prevalence of depression in the terminally ill: effects of diagnostic criteria and symptom threshold judgments. *Am J Psychiatry* 1994; **151**: 537–40.

8 Chochinov HM, Wilson KG, Enns M, Lander S. Depression, hopelessness, and suicidal ideation in the terminally ill. *Psychosomatics.* 1998; **39**: 366–70.

9 Singer PA, Martin DK, Kelner M. Quality end-of-life care: patients' perspectives. *JAMA.* 1999; **281**: 163–8.

10 Chochinov HM, Tataryn D, Dudgeon D, Clinch J. Will to live in the terminally ill. *Lancet.* 1999; **354**: 816–19.

11 Sand L, Strang P. Existential loneliness in a palliative home care setting. *J Palliat Med.* 2006; **9**(6): 1376–87.

12 Proot IM, Abu-Saad HH, Crebolder HFJM *et al.* Vulnerability of family caregivers in terminal palliative care at home: balancing between burden and capacity. *Scand J Caring Sci.* 2003; **17**: 113–21.

13 Chochinov HM. Dignity and the essence of medicine: the A, B, C, and D of dignity conserving care. *BMJ.* 2007; **335**: 184.

14 Nelson CJ, Rosenfeld B, Breitbart W *et al.* Spirituality, religion, and depression in the terminally ill. *Psychosomatics.* 2002; **43**: 213–20.

15 Chao CC, Chen C, Yen M. The essence of spirituality of terminally ill patients. *J Nurs Res.* 2002; **10**: 237–44.

16 Morita T, Tsunoda J, Inoue S *et al.* An exploratory factor analysis of existential suffering in Japanese terminally ill cancer patients. *Psychooncology.* 2000; **9**: 164–8.

17 Kissane DW. Demoralisation: its impact on informed consent and medical care. *Med J Aust.* 2001; **175**: 537–9.

18 Chochinov HM, Wilson KG, Enns M *et al.* Desire for death in the terminally ill. *Am J Psychiatry.* 1995; **152**: 1185–91.

19 Jeffrey D. *Against Physician Assisted Suicide: a palliative care perspective.* Oxford: Radcliffe Publishing; 2008.

20 Breitbart E, Rosenfeld B, Pessin H *et al.* Depression, hopelessness, and desire for hastened death in terminally ill patients with cancer. *JAMA.* 2000; **284**: 2907–11.

21 Wilson KG, Scott JF, Graham ID *et al.* Attitudes of terminally ill patients toward euthanasia and physician-assisted suicide. *Arch Intern Med.* 2000; **160**: 2454–60.

22 Weisman AD. *On Dying and Denying: a psychiatric study of terminality.* New York: Behavioral Publications; 1972.

23 Killminster S. Dignity: not such a useless concept. *J Med Ethics.* 2010; **36**: 160–4.

24 Broyard A. *Intoxicated by my Illness: and other writings on life and death.* New York: Ballantine; 1992.

25 Peabody FW. The care of the patient. *JAMA.* 1927; 88: 876–82.

26 Tolstoy L. *The Death of Ivan Illych.*

27 Dees MK, Vernooij-Dassen MJ, Dekkers WJ *et al.* 'Unbearable suffering': a qualitative study on the perspectives of patients who request assistance in dying. *J Med Ethics.* 2011; **37**: 727–34.

28 Owen R. *Facing the Storm.* London: Routledge; 2011.

29 Williams M, Penman D. *Mindfulness.* London: Piatkus; 2011.

30 Saunders G. *'Love Me or Kill Me': Sarah Kane and the theatre of extremes.* Manchester: Manchester University Press, 2002.

CHAPTER 8

Complexity: *Cloud 9*, Caryl Churchill (1979)

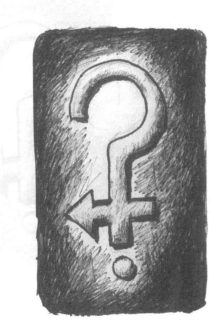

'What are you trying to turn me into?'

Gerry

INTRODUCTION

Caryl Churchill's bleakly comic play *Cloud 9* was devised with the Joint Stock Theatre Company in 1979 and is a play that brilliantly deconstructs social stereotypes, gendered expectations and historical paternalism; it is also a play that presents other problems for us today considering the changed – if, arguably it has changed – social landscape of the 21st century. Like *Blasted*, *Cloud 9* combines naturalistic structures with powerful and experimental image theatre and disorientates the audience with a surreal 'time warp' between Act 1 (set in 19th-century colonial Africa) and Act 2 (set in late 1970s Britain) with almost the same cast of characters present in both.

Though influenced by the Srebrenica massacre, *Blasted*, outside the context of the Leeds hotel, is historically non-specific: we do not know the Soldier's identity or the nature of the civil war that is being fought. In *Cloud 9*, however, the contexts are made explicit – for example the soldier is British, named Billy and stationed in Belfast. Yet we would like to propose that the power structures being examined still have crucial contemporary relevance to clinical assumptions and paternalism in end-of-life care. Before exploring a synopsis of the play, it would be helpful to identify how *Cloud 9* subverts theatrical conventions in terms of the way the characters are represented.

Churchill's play constitutes a formidable and complex challenge for both actors and spectators in its sophisticated, perhaps at times bewildering, use of multi-roling. The feminist critic Micheline Wandor writes: 'the mix in *Cloud 9* […] can arguably "cloud" and weaken the overall strength of the piece'. Churchill specifies that particular roles should be played by actors of a different gender or racial origin, or indeed by objects. For example, Betty in the first act should be played by a man, Joshua, a young Indian boy, should be played by a white actor and Victoria (a young girl) should be 'played' by a doll. While this clearly has comic potential, Churchill's serious purpose is in exploring how we 'construct' other people in accordance with our own experience, expectations or assumptions based on deep-rooted prejudices or historical constructions. As adults we may view the young Victoria as no better than a doll: viewing her as a child we may have limited expectations of her cognitive ability or indeed of her as a 'real' identity – she is thus infantilised to the point of being a non-sentient object. In the opening section of the play, Betty (played a man) remarks of her husband Clive:

> I live for Clive. The whole aim of my life
> Is to be what he looks for in a wife.
> I am a man's creation, as you see,
> And what men want is what I want to be.

Betty is therefore constructed as a man, because she is viewed through the male gaze of particular expectations.

This theatrical construct has significant implications for medical practice. The doctor is trained in physical 'pattern recognition', that is in finding a set of symptoms, based on how the patient presents, that might lead to a diagnosis. But at the same time the doctor may well (perhaps unwittingly) be performing a different and more sinister form of psychological or social 'pattern recognition' in attempting to 'pigeonhole' their social-familial relationships or prescribe how they feel. Just as Churchill in her play shows how characters can be artificially constructed by others, so too can assumptions in a clinical context damage the quality of end-of-life care.

Let us consider the details of the play's narrative before exploring the implications in a clinical context.

PLOT SYNOPSIS

Act 1 is set in British colonial Africa at the end of the 19th century and focuses on one family. The paterfamilias Clive, married to Betty, is having an affair with the widow Mrs Saunders. Clive and Betty's two children, Edward and Victoria, are played by a woman and a dummy respectively. Maud, Clive's mother-in-law, appears both as a confidante to Betty and to emphasise what is ostensibly morally and socially 'correct'. Joshua, the slave boy, played by a white, is seen interacting with various characters and providing a form of a link to the 'outside world' which is depicted by Clive as being cruel and savage.

The first act is characterised by melodramatic language, elements of farce and frequent songs, and explores the convoluted network of affairs and the repressed sexual and racial identities of the characters. We learn that Edward is having sex with the apparently alpha male explorer Harry Bagley. Betty, in turn, lusts after Harry but ends up kissing Ellen (Edward's governess) after revealing this secret to her. Harry also desires a sexual relationship with Clive, but is spurned when the latter expresses his disgust for the idea. The first act closes with a physical struggle between Mrs Saunders, Betty and Clive after which Mrs Saunders is ejected from the family home. There is a small celebration with cake, at which Joshua raises a gun apparently to shoot Clive before blackout.

Act 2 is set in a London park in 1979, but for the characters only 25 years have passed. In this act, with one exception, the characters are played by actors of their own sex. This act is significantly different in mood: the language, while frequently comic, is far more naturalistic than the melodramatic dialogue in Act 1. Only towards the end of the play does the action become increasingly stylised and surreal. We see Betty's children from Act 1, Edward and Victoria, now adult, depicted as their 'natural' sex, as well as being introduced to Lin, a lesbian, and her four-year-old daughter Cathy who is played by a man. This act opens in winter, in a hut in the park, with Lin and Victoria discussing motherhood, and Lin makes a pass at Victoria. Betty arrives and announces she is splitting from her husband. We also learn that Edward is now a gardener for the park and is having a relationship with Gerry. The scene ends with Lin asking Victoria to have sex with her.

The second scene is set in the same park but in spring, with Gerry and Edward who appear to be arguing about their relationship. Gerry, in a long monologue, reveals he has had oral sex with a male stranger in a train compartment. Betty, Martin and Victoria arrive as Cathy plays on a swing. Martin discloses that his marriage to Victoria is in trouble, and he goes on to speak at length of how he champions women and feminism. Lin attempts to persuade Victoria to leave Martin and run away with her; Victoria reveals that her brother, a soldier in Belfast, has been shot dead. Gerry again expresses his lack of interest in his relationship with Edward, which has apparently become stale and domesticated. Edward tells Victoria that he thinks he is lesbian.

The third and penultimate scene in this act takes place in the park in summer. Victoria, Lin and Edward are drunk. The three perform a strange ceremony to restore their status as women and appeal to the Goddesses of ancient times. They then appear to engage in an orgy which Martin interrupts before being dragged into the group. The ghost of Victoria's brother appears and in a foul-mouthed tirade talks of the trauma of being on active service in Northern Ireland. Gerry calls for Edward, and is met with Edward from Act 1 (played by a woman). They appear to have some form of reconciliation and the scene ends with the whole cast singing the song 'Cloud Nine'.

The final scene of the play takes place in the park in late summer and has a plaintive air. Edward tells Gerry he is living with Lin and Victoria and sleeping with them. Gerry appears unfazed by this and invites Edward to dinner. Edward leaves; Harry from Act 1 appears, 'picks up' Gerry and leaves with him. Betty arrives and talks about her frustration with her marriage to Clive and how she has discovered masturbation as a form of release and a way to establish her female identity. Cathy enters with a nosebleed and claims to have been hit and mugged by the boys in the park. Betty and Gerry discuss how it feels to live alone, before Gerry announces he is going to return to Edward and live with him. Clive enters and chides Betty and is disparaging about the decline of the British Empire in Africa.

The play closes with Betty from Act 1 and Betty from Act 2 embracing.

MODERN INTERPRETATIONS AND CULTURAL CONTEXTS

Cloud 9 represents a complex series of interactions where one's personal identity is shaped by others, according to social expectations. In effect, Churchill draws a parallel between the British colonisation of Africa and the way in which notions of gender and sexuality have been 'colonised' by historical patriarchy. Churchill asks us to reconsider our assumptions on sex and race while examining how we as individuals are viewed by society, and the weight that outward appearance carries in terms of how we are treated.

As we indicated in the introduction, some might argue that the specificity of the late 1970s setting undermines any contemporary performance of the play and, indeed, there is a danger that we may be distracted in Churchill's play by the specific historical contexts. 1979 was the year that Margaret Thatcher came to power: Thatcher's dismantling of the welfare state and her lack of engagement with marginalised communities is well-documented. Further, the play certainly has elements of political 'agit-prop' theatre that was popular at the time and may seem dated today. In focusing on notions of colonisation and introducing the ghost of the soldier, Churchill also invokes the Troubles – the bitter civil conflict between the Unionist and Republican communities in Northern Ireland – which were arguably in their darkest and bloodiest stage at the turn of the decade. Nevertheless, we would like to propose that the complexity of *Cloud 9* can provide significant insight in the context of present-day end-of-life care and can teach us valuable lessons about our assumptions and interactions with patients, their families and fellow professionals.

It is worth noting that since *Cloud 9* there have a number of representations of 'hidden' identities in popular culture. In the 1993 neo-noir film *Suture*, which meditates on philosophical issues of identity and appearance, two 'identical' twin brothers are played by a black actor and a white actor, although the other characters do not appear to notice this disparity. David Fincher's *Fight Club* (1997) famously derived its twist from the notion that the two principal characters were actually two 'sides' to one identity, whereas *The Machinist* (2004) offered a variation on this theme: the insomniac machine operator Trevor Reznik is psychologically tortured by a disfigured co-worker who is revealed in the final frames to be a manifestation of his own guilt. Without wishing to oversimplify some of the implications of these ambiguities, what these films and what Churchill's play illuminate is the fundamental schism between who we are and how we are perceived by others.

But the potency of the external image in symbolic terms is also important. Churchill's implicit use of the Troubles as a counterpoint to the 'colonisation' of identity together with her exploration of the power of outward appearance has a powerful resonance with recent events in 'post-conflict' Northern Ireland in its use of symbols. The decision not to fly the Union Jack flag from Belfast City Hall except on certain days sparked violent protests from some sections of the loyalist communities. The political commentator Mark Devenport remarked:

> The former SDLP leader John Hume used to frequently say 'you can't eat a flag'. Ask most Northern Ireland politicians whether they would prefer to spend their time discussing flags or 'bread and butter issues' and they'll tell you the economy every time. Despite that, flags, murals and even the wearing of poppies continue to have the potential to stir sharp divisions.[1]

Yet it is not just the visual symbol that can provoke division, assumption or prejudice. In this chapter we will also explore how employing particular language can have implications for patient–doctor communication.

CLINICAL CONTEXTS

When doctors see patients, they immediately make assumptions based on first impressions. Patients may come to a doctor with a number of seemingly unconnected problems presenting a diagnostic challenge. The first step for a doctor hoping to help a patient is to try to establish a diagnosis. Patients vary in their ability to give a clear account of their symptoms and their story is influenced by their own interpretation and understanding of the meaning of their symptoms. History taking is crucial to reaching a diagnosis since in a majority of cases, the diagnosis is based on the history alone.[2] There are a number of differing ways of reaching a diagnosis; classically, the scientific method of taking a history of the patient's symptoms and then examining the patient for signs of disease leads to the formation of a list of diagnostic possibilities.[3] There may be investigations planned to elucidate which of the differential diagnoses is the most likely to be correct. This deductive method may be contrasted with pattern recognition. Here the practitioner relies on their experience, rapidly reaching a diagnosis based on intuition.

In clinical practice the doctor listens to the patient's story; they may recognise quickly a cluster of symptoms and leap to the diagnosis (pattern recognition) or there may be a longer period of questions and answers before a few diagnostic possibilities emerge which may then be tested further.[4]

CASE HISTORY: PAULINE

Pauline, aged 48, has a three-month history of increasing fatigue, loss of appetite and weight loss. She has had no pain. Over the past four weeks she has become increasingly jaundiced. Her stools are pale and her urine is dark. On examination her liver is enlarged with a hard edge. The doctor diagnoses pancreatic cancer with spread to the liver by 'pattern recognition'. This may be confirmed by the 'deductive method' of organising blood tests and scans to confirm the diagnosis.

Pattern recognition may of course lead to the doctor jumping to the wrong conclusions because this intuitive reasoning involves making assumptions. The problem is made more acute by frequent media coverage of doctors' mistakes, leading to added pressure in diagnostic situations. Doctors are unhappy with uncertainty: yet uncertainty is one factor that is inevitable in a clinical context. Let us take a different example where an assumption has more serious consequences.

CASE HISTORY: KATHY

Kathy, aged 28, comes to her GP with central chest pain which she notices is worse when she plays tennis. Kathy is overweight and a worrier so the GP assumes, because she is so young, that heart disease can be safely excluded as a diagnostic possibility. He reassures her that the pain was probably indigestion and prescribes antacids with dietary advice. Three weeks later Kathy is admitted to hospital following a collapse. Investigations reveals coronary artery disease which requires triple by-pass surgery. The GP was reasonable to use pattern recognition which led him to disregard a cardiac cause for her pain because at that age, in the absence of other risk factors, ischaemic heart disease is very rare.

While tackling diagnostic assumptions is one challenge facing the doctor, attempting to break down assumptions about what patients want is far more difficult. In complex situations, such as end-of-life care, doctors and other healthcare professionals seek to clarify the problems by trying to simplify issues. Pattern recognition is one way of doing this; using diagnostic algorithms and care pathways are other ways of making sense from an uncertain complex situation. These methods involve the doctor making assumptions and reaching decisions about general probabilities rather than achieving a more thorough understanding of the patient as an individual.

Assumptions and pattern recognition may be an integral part of reaching a clinical diagnosis, but they can lead to mistakes if extended to the other (arguably more important) parts of a patient's life. When assumptions are made about a patient on the basis of a doctor's prejudices and values then stereotyping becomes likely.

Clive's paternalism (and related hypocrisy) dominates the first act of *Cloud 9* as he maintains an iron grip on his household. Further, Clive's family at a microcosmic level represents the unyielding and blinkered traditions of the British Empire. Assumption is at the heart of Clive's world-view, and dissent or difference is met with belligerence. While Betty has some form of catharsis at the end of the play – signified by her embrace of her 'historical' counterpart

– Clive is left in a position of limbo. He feels betrayed and let down by his wife who has behaved in a way that is out of step with his expectations.

There are examples in a clinical context of end-of-life care where assumptions may be made which can result in grouping individuals into categories or stereotypes. Assumptions about a patient may include:

- 'She is a poor historian.'
- 'He would lose all hope and give up if we disclosed the true diagnosis.'
- 'She only has a few weeks to live.'
- 'She must want to fight the cancer.'
- 'We must not give up on treatment.'
- 'He would not want cardiopulmonary resuscitation.'
- 'She is demented so she can't make any decisions.'

Assumptions are made about families:

- 'The husband blames us for her illness.'
- 'They just want her out of the house.'
- 'She's a nurse; she should look after her husband.'
- 'They can't want to sleep together; he is far too ill.'
- 'They are from an Asian background so the family will want to do all the caring.'

Assumptions can be made about the place of care:

- 'Hospital is the best place to be when you are ill.'
- 'You are dying so a hospice would be best.'
- 'Everyone wants to be at home to die.'
- 'No one wants to die on their own.'

Healthcare professionals make assumptions about each other:

- 'He is a surgeon so avoids talking about death and dying.'
- 'Palliative care should be started when all treatments have finished.'
- 'Hospices care only for the dying.'
- 'Nurses can deal with the emotional problems.'

Stereotyping risks degenerating into racism, sexism, elitism and other negative behaviours which categorise people in an unfair way. A reliance on stereotypes means that people stop looking for, or attending to, information which conflicts with the stereotypes. In a clinical context this has an important implication; doctors need to get to know their patients and team members as individuals.

CASE HISTORY: JIM

Jim is a 70-year-old man with advanced bowel cancer and is in a hospice for his terminal care as he lives on his own. His doctors feel that discussing a Do Not Attempt Cardiopulmonary Resuscitation Order (DNACPR) is not necessary because it would be futile and they assume this discussion would cause Jim unnecessary distress. Jim's pain proves difficult to control and one night a nurse sitting with him asks him if he is worried about dying. Jim tells her that it is not dying that worries him, but he is terrified that the doctors might try to resuscitate him. He is too frightened to raise the issue with his doctors. When the nurse reassures him that she will pass on his wishes to the medical team and that they would definitely not attempt cardiopulmonary resuscitation in the event of his death Jim is relieved, his requirements for analgesics drops and his pain becomes straightforward to control.

When assumptions are linked to stereotyping and paternalism then the patient becomes removed from decision making and his autonomy is threatened. Paternalism often springs from good motives, a desire to help the patient and to avoid causing distress. However, patients are tougher than doctors give them credit for. The ethical path for a doctor is to avoid making assumptions and instead to check out their ideas with the patient in a sensitive manner. In complex end-of-life decisions the GMC warns doctors against taking a personal view about a patient's quality of life and to avoid making judgements based on assumptions about the healthcare needs of the elderly or the disabled.[5] Complex history taking skills may only be learned through experience and reflective practice. It is by reflecting on our assumptions that we question whether we have listened to the patient's view or paternalistically forced our choices onto them.

But the dangers of assumptions and stereotyping are only one part of the complexity of *Cloud 9*. We would like to look at the narrative of the play in more detail to identify some key dynamics that may help us to understand related tensions in end-of-life care, with a particular focus on pressures that the characters face. We may, for example, find Clive a bullying and unpleasant character, but he is a product of his social and historical context. If we strive to be good doctors, it is important for us to be aware of these pressures in order to manage them effectively.

From the outset, Churchill establishes colonial Africa as a place rife with suspicion, secrets and intrigue. But why does the playwright choose this specific setting for the characters to grapple with their identities? We might argue that the Victorian context suggests the necessity to 'keep up appearances' at all times within a very rigid social hierarchy that is both heteronormative and openly racist. Clive's opening comment serves to establish himself as the uber-masculine father figure that is socially dominant:

> CLIVE: This is my family. Though far from home
> We serve the Queen wherever we may roam
> I am father to the natives here,
> And father to my family so dear.
> [He presents BETTY. She is played by a man.]
> My wife is all I dreamt a wife should be,
> And everything she is she owes to me.

The deliberately laboured, trite rhymes and the incongruity of Betty's physical sex sets Clive up as a one-dimensional, comic figure who is blind to any nuances of difference in identity.

Consultants may be assumed to be the leaders of the multidisciplinary team, but effective team-working challenges this stereotyping. The nurse, occupational therapist, psychologist, social worker, district nurse or GP may be the key professional in any particular case and so take a lead role in coordinating the team. It is important in any team that every individual feels comfortable with other team members questioning their decisions or acting as the patient's advocate. Such input to team discussions should not be perceived as criticism of the professional but rather adding valuable perspectives into the care of the patient. If consultants or GPs establish strict hierarchies or are perceived as unapproachable, or even 'scary', by other team members then patient care is impaired.

Doctors who isolate themselves by seeming to know all the answers, never admitting vulnerability or being reluctant to seek advice, put themselves under enormous pressure. This pressure may be increased by a patient's expectation that the doctor will have some other treatment to offer or that he will be able to solve all their problems. Pressure may come from a society which can expect doctors to behave in ways that may conflict with their own values. For instance, in the recent debate about the legalisation of assisted suicide and euthanasia, it is often assumed that doctors would be willing to take part if the law is passed.

Recently a man with locked-in syndrome appealed to the courts to allow doctors to assist him to die as he felt his life was undignified and had no quality.[6] The courts refused his appeal and this precipitated the media to call for changes in the law on euthanasia and assisted suicide. This situation is highly complex; human sympathy for a distressed individual may well assume 'of course his life should be ended, if that's what he wants'. However, more considered reflection of this assumption takes into account the broader implications of changing the law for everyone on the basis of one difficult case.[7] A change in the law would involve a paradigm shift in the nature and ethos of medical practice. Doctors have autonomy, too, and other vulnerable patients might be put at risk if doctors were permitted to kill. A true liberal concept of autonomy does not give people an unbridled right to do whatever they wish but places a responsibility on them to consider the effects of their choices on others in society. Laws cannot be made for exceptional cases, since they function as imperfect tools for protecting the majority.

In the clinical context doctors working within a hierarchy can feel a pressure to keep up appearances. This can be manifest by a junior doctor's reluctance to question the decisions of a senior consultant in case she is perceived as being critical. Patients can also be intimidated by doctors whom they perceive as 'busy' or too important to bother with their possibly trivial worries. Paternalistic behaviour by the doctor is another way of maintaining the hierarchy . . . 'I know what is best for you'. Doctors can use jargon, oversimplifying the situation, such as 'Just pop up on the couch and slip off your clothes, I want to examine your chest', which can humiliate patients.

Sometimes consultants can use sarcasm to humiliate students in front of colleagues 'My granny knows more medicine than you.' Such unprofessional behaviour risks students becoming bullies when they, in time, become consultants.

In Chapter 6 we explored the notion of 'concealment' in *All My Sons*. In Miller's naturalistic drama, the 'buried' truth serves as a catalyst to the action, and precipitates the final tragedy of Joe Keller's suicide. In *Cloud 9* this 'concealment' is realised in a different dimension through the use of actors that differ from the race or gender of the characters they portray. But while in *All My Sons* the uncovering of the truth takes place over the course of the narrative, for an audience watching *Cloud 9* these 'concealed' identities are immediately apparent.

Concealment and dishonesty are explored in detail in Chapter 6, but it is worth pointing out that patients often take time to assess their doctor before divulging the true reason for their consultation. In the example of Jim discussed earlier he was unwilling to discuss his fears with his doctors but found that he could talk more openly to a nurse. Patients will often give doctors a cue, in a throwaway remark, and if the doctor misses this emotional cue the patient will often not raise it with them again.

For instance, a patient with advanced cancer may say to her doctor, 'Doctor, I am worried about the pain in my hip.'

The doctor may respond in two different ways, each of which will have a very different outcome for the patient's care. Either he could say, 'Please tell me more about the pain, is it relieved by the painkillers I prescribed?'

Or, he might say, 'I want to help with the pain, but first could you please tell me a bit more about what you are worried about?'

In the first instance the doctor and patient will have a medical discussion about types and doses of painkillers. The second response will give the patient an opportunity to discuss their real concerns which are probably the reason why their pain is not relieved by the analgesics. Part of the skill of good communication in end-of-life care is for a doctor to see beyond the patient's brave face and to beware of making assumptions.

But why do the characters conceal their true identities? And why, in Act 2, are almost all of the characters played by actors of the 'correct' gender or race? One clue may be the different environments in the two acts. The Victorian setting in Act 1 stifles the characters, whereas the park in Act 2 is a place of exploration and play.

In the clinical context the patient may receive care in a variety of environments; their own home, a hospital ward, outpatient department, hospice or nursing home. The patient's behaviour can be influenced by these different surroundings. Generally, people feel most relaxed in their own homes and this is one reason why home visiting of terminally ill patients is such an integral part of a doctor's care. It often seems that the presence of the doctor and their continued interest in the patient, evidenced by their willingness to visit them in their home, enables the patient and family to cope without hospital admission for end-of-life care.

TIME, COMPASSION AND JUSTICE

Cloud 9 makes us re-examine our thoughts about time. In a strict scientific sense time is usually thought of as the uniform continuous time of Newton.[9] This view does not take into account time as a changeable concept, time as it is actually lived. Waiting two hours in an outpatient clinic for the result of a blood test before receiving chemotherapy can seem a great deal longer than two hours spent on the golf course.

Time has become a precious commodity in healthcare and doctors effectively have to ration the time they spend with patients. Patients value their time with physicians and generally want more of it.[10] However, it appears that doctors seem to be working harder, seeing more patients but spending less time with them. Many doctors are spending more time on administrative duties.[10]

A 'scarcity paradigm' permeates the culture of the NHS.[14] The most important commodity which is in short supply is time. The consequence of the managerial emphasis on reducing time spent with patients and cutting the time patients spend in hospitals is that the emotional and psychological elements of care, such as compassion, are rendered impractical and devalued.[11] The current culture in many hospitals is that nurses and doctors are so busy that compassionate care has become an unaffordable luxury. Dissenters who do spend time sitting with patients and listening to them are regarded as 'slow workers' or 'too talkative'.[11] The scarcity paradigm not only causes patients to receive less compassionate care but it contributes to burnout in doctors and nurses. Healthcare professionals want to provide care which is competent and compassionate and when they are prevented from doing this they feel stressed.[12] The need to bring compassion back into care has recently been recognised by the Chief Nursing Officer for England with the launch of *Compassion in Practice*.[13]

Shortage of time creates an ethical dilemma between a duty to be fair (justice) and to provide high-quality care (compassion). Compassion, we have argued in this book, is the moral response to the patient in need, most particularly to dying patients. The rationing dilemma is often presented as one where Justice is pitted against Compassion. In other words, it is argued that if a doctor gives one patient extra time other patients will be put at risk. In this model Justice will trump Compassion and the patient will receive less high-quality care and doctors and nurses will be at risk of burnout.[14]

However, a counter-argument can be made that if justice and compassion are not seen as moral opposites but instead compassion is seen as an integral part of justice then a different model emerges. In this way a sense of justice assumes a personal value. Doctors and nurses who respond to a patient's needs can then be seen as having a sense of justice.[14] Compassion can play an ethical role in motivating morally justified acts which can be moderated by a linked duty of fairness. In this way of looking at personal justice there is no chance of compassion being ignored in the delivery of healthcare.[15] Furthermore, seeing compassion as a response to injustice enhances respect for patient dignity and legitimises advocacy on behalf of the patient.[15]

MODEL OF COMPLEXITY

The model illustrates some of the factors which interact in the individual patient to generate complex problems. These may be physical, psychological, spiritual, emotional or ethical challenges encountered in end-of-life care and are often a complex mix of several domains. Guidelines and evidence-based medicine (EBM) may help to clarify complexity, but the physician needs to remember that EBM is based on generality and the patient is an individual. The experienced physician will combine both an EBM and personal approach to patient care.

CONCLUSIONS

In this chapter we have focused on the complexity of the issues within palliative care. Decisions need to take account of not only physical factors of the disease but psychological, social and spiritual issues must also be taken into

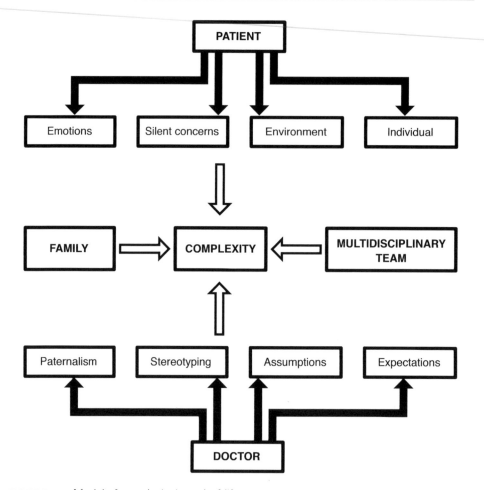

FIGURE 8.1 Model of complexity in end-of-life care

consideration.[8] This places an obligation on healthcare professionals to listen to patients and to develop individual treatment plans which take account of both the patient's and their families' views. It is tempting in these most complex situations to make assumptions and to react intuitively when more careful reflection uncovers a far more complex problem.

We have discussed how compassion in clinical care is threatened by the scarcity paradigm.[14] By seeing compassion as an integral part of being fair (Justice) to patients professionals can feel empowered to spend time with patients and to act as their advocates to counter organisational cultures which devalue compassion.

REFERENCES

1 Devenport M. Belfast police defend City Hall flag riot response. BBC News. 4 December 2012. Available online at www.bbc.co.uk/news/uk-northern-ireland-20594139 (accessed 16 January 2013).

2 Bosk CL. Occupational rituals in patient management. *N Engl J Med.* 1980; **303**: 71–6.

3 Baerheim A. The diagnostic process in general practice: has it a two-phase structure? *J Fam Pract.* 2001; **18**(3): 243–5.

4 Sackett DL, Haynes RB, Guvatt GH *et al. Clinical Epidemiology.* Boston: Little, Brown and Co.; 1991. pp. 3–18.

5 GMC. *Treatment and Care Towards the End of Life: good practice in decision-making.* Available online at: www.gmc-uk.org/guidance/ethical guidance (accessed 17 August 2012).

6 Toynbee P. Would you be happy to live like Tony Nicklinson? *The Guardian.* 17 August 2012.

7 Wollaston S. Assisted dying: the harm in helping. Comment is free. *The Guardian.* 17 August 2012. Available online at: www.guardian.co.uk/commentisfree/2012/aug/17/assisted-suicide-causes-harm? (accessed 19 August 2012).

8 Munday DF. Complexity theory and palliative care. *Palliat Med.* 2003; **17**: 308–9.

9 Kern S. Time and medicine. *Ann Intern Med.* 2000; **132**: 3–9.

10 Morrison I. The future of physicians' time. *Ann Intern Med.* 2000; **132**: 80–4.

11 Heath I. Humane decisions. *Nurs Times.* 1997; **93**: 26–7.

12 Lutzen K. Moral stress. *Nurs Ethics.* 2003; **10**: 312–22.

13 Department of Health. *Compassion in Practice.* Available online at: www.dh.gov.uk/health/2012/12/nursing-vision/ (accessed 16 January 2013).

14 Maxwell B. Just compassion: implications for the ethics of the scarcity paradigm in clinical health care. *J Med Ethics.* 2009; **35**: 219–23.

15 Kristjansson K. *Justice and Desert-based Emotions.* Aldershot: Ashgate; 2006.

CHAPTER 9

Culture: *Behzti*, Gurpreet Kaur Bhatti (2004)

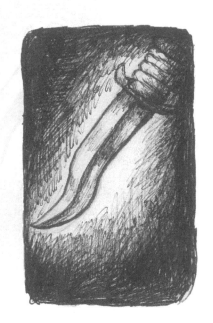

INTRODUCTION

After Sarah Kane's *Blasted*, perhaps no other play in recent British history has attracted as much press controversy as Gurpreet Kaur Bhatti's *Behzti (Dishonour)*. The play, which displays rape and murder in the most sacred part of a Sikh temple, ran for only one week at the Birmingham Repertory Theatre before being closed down due to violent protest, damage to the theatre's glass façade and death threats sent to the young playwright. The decision to drop the piece was roundly condemned by the press; *The Daily Telegraph*'s reaction was typical of the general media commentary surrounding *Behzti*:

> It is understandable that those who have had their religion insulted are outraged; but only as long as that outrage remains within the bounds of the law. . . . The response to offensive art or rhetoric shouldn't be violence (or a criminal conviction, as per the proposed law against religious hatred). If you are outraged by the Birmingham play, the response is simple: use lawful means of protest or just don't buy a ticket. What we have instead is a play that has been censored and a playwright in hiding for fear of her life.[1]

Response from the Sikh community was mixed. Some supported the writer, others, such as Mohan Singh, a Sikh community leader, felt that the play was blasphemous and mocking to Sikhism: 'When they're doing a play about a Sikh priest raping somebody inside a gurdwara, would any religion take it?'[2]

Many felt the play had been misunderstood. Yasmin Wilde, who played the rape victim in the premiere, commented: 'The message of the play isn't "isn't religion awful". It's about how human frailty can take you away from what's true about your religion.'[3]

The key issue for many was the setting of the play. Members of the Sikh community suggested that if the rape and murder (which take place offstage) was set in a Sikh community centre rather than a temple the play could be performed. Bhatti refused to bow to their demands, although she did make slight alterations to the script.

While it would be glib to suggest that the controversy surrounding the play was short-lived, Bhatti was not charged with incitement to racial hatred – as was suggested at the time – and the play has been published, is widely taught at university and was performed as a rehearsed reading at London's Soho theatre in 2010 without incident.

The columnist Robert Sharp, who attended the reading, remarked: 'Six years after its abortive first production, *Behzti* still feels current and relevant. The actors turned in a robust delivery with very little time to rehearse, as if they were picking up where they left off. They have reinforced the artistic case for a proper revival.'[4]

SYNOPSIS

It is important to note that *Behzti* is a play that is carefully structured and sub-
divided into scenes with specific titles. Obviously, an audience will be unaware
of these subdivisions, but the ordered structure creates a quality of ominous
logic and process – perhaps reflecting the way orthodoxy can undermine a
community as well as uniting it.

Min, a young Sikh woman, must care for her mother, Balbir, who is house-
bound. In the first scene we are shown that Balbir is rude, bullying and selfish.
While Min appears respectful of Sikh traditions, Balbir dismisses them with
foul language and implies that Min should make an effort with her appearance
in order to attract men. Min and Balbir are preparing to visit the Sikh temple
for the evening ceremony. We are then introduced to Elvis, a young black man
in his twenties who is Balbir's professional 'carer'. Balbir is flirtatious then abusive to Elvis, who does not rise to Balbir's provocation. Min and Elvis look after
Balbir until she falls asleep, then the pair have a moment of intimacy and discuss the possibility of going out on a date together, after which Elvis convinces
Min to tell him about the ritual in the Sikh temple. Elvis leaves and Min wakes
Balbir, who in turn tells Min that she doesn't want to visit the temple that evening before calling Min a 'thickhead' and racially abusing Elvis.

With Balbir continuing to insult Min, Min tapes up Balbir's mouth and ties
her wrists and only removes them when Balbir agrees to put her faith both in
God and in Elvis.

Balbir goes on to reminisce about her own wedding, and the traditions of
the past, before bringing up the topic of Mr Sandhu, a wealthy senior member
of the Sikh community who is refurbishing the Gurdwara. Balbir insists that
Mr Sandhu has 'taken a great interest' in both herself and in Min, and then
reveals that she has contacted Sandhu who in turn has put Min on a 'list' to
match her up with a wealthy husband. Min is angered by her mother's actions
and refuses to see Sandhu. This infuriates the scheming Balbir who apparently
cannot understand why a 'bloody horse' like Min does not want this 'opportunity'. The mother then tells Min that it is Min's father who has left them destitute
and again orders her daughter to see Mr Sandhu. Min refuses but agrees instead
to visit the Gurdwara with her mother briefly.

The next scene, set in the Gurdwara, is made up of a series of illuminated
spaces within the temple where we are introduced to further characters in the

play. The first is Giana Jaswant, an elderly priest who sits and listens to 'hypnotic Sikh religious music' and waves a horsehair stick in time. The next is Mr Sandhu, who is shown wearing a cheap suit, in his office, throwing darts at a Sikh calendar and rewarding himself with sweets. The sense of religious transgression is emphasised by the fact that we are told that his turban lies on the desk.

The following illuminated scene introduces Polly Dhodhar and Teetee Parmar, two women in late middle age who are stealing from the shoe-rack in the Gurdwara. The pair exchange friendly banter about shoes and gossip about various figures in their community. Teetee reveals that Mr Sandhu is planning an extension to the Gurdwara and that her son Billoo has been asked to take on the project. Polly slyly 'jokes' that she would like to invite Billoo to dinner, which prompts an angry response from Teetee who grabs her and tells her to leave her son alone. Their conversation is interrupted by Giani Jaswant who walks past, apparently distracted. Polly and Teetee are deferential to Jaswant, who is evidently mentally confused and talks gibberish to the women. The women discuss Jaswant's apparent drug use and go to leave to work in the kitchen when they are interrupted by the arrival of Balbir, Min and Elvis.

In the first part of the scene, Balbir and Teetee reminisce fondly about Teetee's wedding. There is an awkward moment where Elvis is introduced, with Balbir insisting that he is her carer and not Min's boyfriend. The older women again talk about their shared past, particularly their apparently impoverished childhood in a run-down environment where they experienced racial abuse. Polly and Teetee seem kind towards Min but Balbir interrupts their compliments by telling them it is 'time to think of the future'. Polly and Teetee talk about their current familial situations, with Polly telling Balbir that her husband has recently died. The women discuss their apparently comfortable work situations and praise Mr Sandhu for contributing to the life of the Gurdwara, although they are clearly slightly unnerved by Sandhu's decision to make the erratic Jaswant a priest (the scene cuts for a moment to show Jaswant eating while sitting on the toilet).

Balbir next reveals to Teetee that she knows of Mr Sandhu's 'list' and that she is keen to get Min an arranged marriage and that the 'old ways never did [them] any harm'. Min and Elvis enter, with the women ensuring that Elvis has his head covered – the only thing they have is a woman's scarf which Elvis reluctantly puts on. The group argue about whether Balbir is able to go for a walk, leaving Min 'fearful' in the tense situation.

We then find Polly and Elvis together, rummaging through an Indian trunk to find a headscarf for Elvis to wear. Polly asks whether Elvis has a girlfriend and seems generally inquisitive about the young man. Once Elvis has a scarf on, Polly moves closer to him and we are told that the moment 'sizzles with sexual tension'. They seem to be about to kiss, before Elvis breaks away and leaves guiltily.

We are then shown Balbir and Teetee 'preparing for Mr Sandhu'. Balbir is at pains to talk about how she has engineered a future meeting between Min and Mr Sandhu. Teetee is appreciative, but Balbir becomes aggressive, claiming that she has spent her life looking after other people. Teetee responds 'jokingly', causing Balbir to say that she herself was joking. There is an uneasy moment, before Teetee suggests that they prepare themselves for entering Mr Sandhu's room.

The next scene takes place inside the Gurdwara and comprises an encounter between Min and the elderly cleric Giani Jaswant. Min is unsettled by the enigmatic man, and cautiously asks him questions. Giani in turn tells Min a transformative story about a 'bedraggled man' who eventually finds a safe community and his faith. Min is impressed by the story but Giani falls silent and will not answer Min's questions. Elvis enters, looking for Balbir. Min is still clearly overwhelmed by Giani's stories and asks Elvis to sing a hymn while she washes up.

Scene 5 is pivotal in the action of the play. Balbir meets with Mr Sandhu in the Gurdwara to discuss the list, yet Mr Sandhu seems distracted and talks about a couple that Balbir knew, much to Balbir's impatience. Finally, Balbir manages to convince Mr Sandhu to talk about his 'list' and brings up the subject of Min. Mr Sandhu appears interested at first but then digresses again and tells Balbir that his wife committed suicide. He appears almost comically detached from her death, and Balbir is bewildered. Mr Sandhu asks Balbir if Min is a virgin; when Balbir affirms this he remarks that this is a 'plus point'. Finally, he tells Balbir he is willing to meet Min, but she must first go and pray.

Min and Elvis are seen washing up in the Gurdwara kitchen, where Giani Jaswant is sleeping. Min is in high spirits and sings a Christian song, and Elvis responds by singing a spiritual song of his own. He asks Min to teach him a Sikh song, which she does. She tells Elvis she is happy in the Gurdwara, but Elvis is a little unsettled: we infer that he feels Min doesn't have a social life outside of her Sikh faith. Elvis then tells her how he spends most nights in the pub, occasionally being asked to sing on the stage. At Min's request he sings another song, Bob Marley's 'One Drop'. Giani wakes up and joins in the singing, causing Elvis to be embarrassed. Min apologises for Elvis singing a Christian song, but Elvis denies he is a Christian. Giani tells them that 'there is no Christian or Hindu or Muslim or Jew or Buddhist or Rastafarian or Sikh', which surprises the young couple. When pressed on this, Giani states that he has found spiritual insight from visiting the Notting Hill Carnival, and exits, leaving Min and Elvis confused. Elvis appears to want to say something romantic to Min, but is cut short when Balbir enters to take Min away to Mr Sandhu. Elvis wants to go with them, but Balbir refuses, telling him this a special time for mother and daughter. Elvis asks them not to go, but they leave for Mr Sandhu regardless.

Mr Sandhu is shown playing darts again, and talking to Teetee. We learn that Teetee's husband has gone to India, but Teetee doesn't appear to care, much to Mr Sandhu's disapproval. Teetee raises the subject of her son Billoo and asks Mr Sandhu if Billoo might work on the extension for the Gurdwara. Mr Sandhu is sceptical at first and asks Teetee about Billoo's background and training. He finally agrees, but the atmosphere turns sinister when he asks Teetee if he can 'count on' her. Teetee nervously agrees.

The action moves to the men's toilets at the Gurdwara. Elvis asks Giani Jaswant for his advice: clearly he is in love with Min but, as he explains the situation, he does not realise that Polly is present but remains unseen. Polly assumes Elvis's declaration of love applies to herself and becomes excited, jumping up and down and spraying herself with deodorant. Giani seems confused again at Elvis's request for help, and leaves. Polly emerges and, delighted with Elvis's 'confession', kisses him on the lips. Elvis is horrified and realises how Polly has misunderstood. He claims he has 'spoilt it all' and that he is a 'big bag of nothing'.

The next scene opens with Mr Sandhu praying. Elvis is talking to Polly in the kitchen and trying to apologise for his behaviour. Polly remains resolute: she suggests that the two of them should run away and make love with music blaring. They kiss again, but Elvis is clearly feeling guilty. Polly continues to press Elvis and declares her feelings for him. Elvis counters by telling her that he wasn't talking about her when he spoke with Giani. The truth dawns on Polly, who, enraged, starts to physically attack Elvis. Teetee interrupts the fight and asks what is happening. Elvis tries to explain, Polly shows her contempt for Elvis as someone who is 'not what he seems'. Teetee grabs Elvis's face and tells him that the Sikh rules are above the law of the land, and that he should be careful. He goes to leave, and Polly 'furiously' quotes Sikh scripture at him, reminding him of the power of their God.

Elvis approaches Giani and begs him not to disclose his love for Min. Giani responds by telling Elvis he must be honest with Min and declare his feelings to her and cites the Guru Granth Sahib. Elvis then joins the congregation, where Polly and Teetee complain about the quality of the sacrament, the *parshad*. Elvis causes embarrassment by sitting in the wrong part of the Gurdwara. The scene ends with Giani chanting scripture to the congregation.

The next scene is entitled 'Wrongdoing'. Min stands in Mr Sandhu's office. She becomes curious about the items on Mr Sandhu's desk, and finds a Bee Gees CD. She begins to hum 'How Deep is Your Love' and dances with a kirpan (the sacred Sikh dagger). Mr Sandhu enters and Min freezes in embarrassment. Mr Sandhu claims he has seen Min in the park when she was child, riding her bike. Min says she doesn't remember. Min asks Mr Sandhu about the CD and is told that the music 'keeps him going', after which Mr Sandhu breaks down and bursts into tears.

Mr Sandhu is comforted by Min, who offers him a tissue. He then asks if Min came to see the 'list', but she replies simply that she came because her mother wanted her to. Min is then asked if she has someone 'inside her heart', but Min will only give the first letter of Elvis's name. The conversation turns to Tej, Min's absent father. Mr Sandhu reveals that he was in love with Tej, and that Min had stumbled upon him and Tej kissing. Min is thunderstruck and claims not to remember. Mr Sandhu is inconsolable and reaffirms his love for Tej. Min, upset, tries to leave but Mr Sandhu grabs her. Min's screaming merges with the chants of the congregation.

The service comes to a close and Elvis, alone, begins to sing in Min's honour. When the traumatised Min arrives, Elvis declares his love for her in a poetic fashion. The dazed Min rebuffs his advances, but Elvis persists. Min angrily tells him that he is simply 'home care' and nothing more. Elvis needs his sheet signed for his work with Balbir. Min finally tells him to stay still and she will get his sheet signed. As she turns to leave, we are told that she reveals a 'terrifying' patch of blood on her rear.

Balbir, Teetee and Polly are in the kitchen of the Gurdwara. Balbir is elated in her anticipation of the announcement of Min's engagement, but the others are downbeat and distracted. Giani enters in a similarly plaintive mood. The group briefly discuss Elvis's 'misbehaviour'. Polly asks Giani 'never to speak of this again', but Giani replies enigmatically and leaves. Balbir instigates a discussion on Min's wedding, having claimed that her daughter has been 'conjugated' to a bachelor on Mr Sandhu's 'list'. Balbir stirs the women up by claiming that they will be a key part of the wedding and asks for their help. When they agree, Balbir becomes even more excited, saying that it will be 'like the old days'. The trio sing a bawdy song, but are interrupted by Min's arrival.

The women notice the stain on Min's clothes and assume she is menstruating. The atmosphere turns sinister as Balbir, Polly and Teetee accuse her of bringing 'dishonour' to the Gurdwara and begin to verbally abuse her before instigating a physical attack on her. Having been assaulted by Polly and Teetee, Balbir is invited to strike Min, which she does as the others call her a 'dirty bitch'.

Mr Sandhu enters and orders the women to stop the attack. He slyly asserts that he has a plan that would put a 'silver lining' on the situation. Balbir appears intrigued but is forced to leave to empty her bladder. After she has gone, Min screams for her and tells the group that Mr Sandhu has raped her. Teetee orders Min to 'apologise' for the rape, but Min stands her ground and angrily denounces Mr Sandhu, claiming that God knows what he has done. Mr Sandhu begins to cry and offer an 'explanation' that the rape can be blamed on Min for being a 'Temptress'. Min attempts to escape but is restrained and attacked by Teetee who demands again that she apologise. Min quietly does so, before Teetee releases Min and spits at Mr Sandhu's feet, saying, 'She's yours'. Teetee exits, leaving Min to the mercy of Mr Sandhu.

Mr Sandhu asks if she is hurt, before launching into a speech about being incited to rape her because she reminded him of her father whom he again asserts he loved. He gives Min the Bee Gees CD but Min is furious and accuses him of lying and having raped before. Mr Sandhu acknowledges this and leaves. Min, physically and emotionally drained, attempts to sing a Bee Gees song but cannot and slumps to the floor.

Teetee returns, telling Min that marrying Mr Sandhu is a 'sacrifice' that will benefit everyone. Balbir enters and asks Min if Mr Sandhu has 'popped the question'. When Min replies in the affirmative, her mother tries to reassure her that Mr Sandhu will die soon, leaving her a generous will and the chance to remarry. Min simply tells Balbir that she must remember to sign Elvis's home care sheet. Balbir unconvincingly insists that 'everything will be alright'. Teetee says 'it's finished' and offers Min a cup of tea, but Min strikes her arm and sends the tea flying across the room before leaving.

Teetee and Balbir are left alone to talk. Balbir, delusional, tells Teetee that Min has been searching for a fish, but has caught a whale and muses on the prospect of asking her future son-in-law for a 'list' of his own. Teetee flatly tells Balbir that 'there is no list' and verbally abuses Balbir for her stupidity. Balbir, becoming increasingly agitated, asks Teetee naively why Mr Sandhu would promise a non-existent 'list'. Teetee tells her that it is so Mr Sandhu can rape girls and sometimes boys that come to see him. When Balbir challenges Teetee and asks how she knows, Teetee responds by telling her that she herself was raped by Mr Sandhu. Balbir is incredulous and asks why Teetee beat and insulted Min. Teetee claims she was 'doing her duty' and reminds Balbir that she, too, hit her daughter. Balbir pathetically lunges at Teetee but misses her and falls to the floor. Teetee says she is going home, and Balbir cries out for her, asking what will happen to Min, to which Teetee replies 'the same as the rest of us' and leaves with Balbir sobbing on the floor.

In a horribly mundane contrast to the previous scene, we now see Mr Sandhu in his office with Polly and Giani, flicking through a paint pamphlet and discussing with the others suitable colours for the Gurdwara extension. Mr Sandhu becomes suspicious of Giani's erratic behaviour and asks him if he has been taking drugs. Giani admits he has, in order to find spiritual transcendence. Mr Sandhu becomes angry and insists that he has saved Giani from his demons and asks Giani to thank him for this. We infer from their conversation that Giani has been involved with a woman of whom Mr Sandhu disapproved and that the woman is now in prison. Giani claims to have a vision of a woman 'snogging a black boy' and points at Polly who is clearly terrified that her secret will be revealed. Giani leaves and Mr Sandhu tells Polly that she is no longer a part of the Gurdwara refurbishing committee.

Teetee enters and Mr Sandhu passes Polly a notepad and pen, asking her to take a dictation. This turns out to be a letter to a building firm asking them to take on the contract for the extension. Teetee realises that Mr Sandhu has ignored her son's request to take on the building work and has instead chosen a non-Sikh company. Mr Sandhu asks Polly to bring him some tea and Polly exits, leaving a traumatised and angry Teetee to face her tormentor.

Mr Sandhu tells Teetee that the building work 'is not for Indians' and sometimes they must 'defer to the greater authority of our white brothers'. This enrages Teetee who tells Mr Sandhu she will go to the police and report the rapes. Mr Sandhu calmly tells her that there are witnesses to her beating of Min and that no one will believe her if she accuses him of rape. Teetee's rage increases as she pushes Mr Sandhu to the ground and seizes the kirpan, the Sikh dagger, and holds it over Mr Sandhu's body. She goes on to cite scripture that focuses on the Sikhs rising up violently against their oppressors. Mr Sandhu is terrified and begs Teetee to stop. Balbir enters, tells Teetee to stop and takes the kirpan from Teetee's hand. The lights fade.

The final scene of the play is entitled 'Resurrection'. A bedraggled Min stumbles towards Elvis with his signed home care sheet. Elvis asks her what has happened and she tells him she has had an 'accident'. Elvis carries Min into the men's toilets where they encounter Giani who is washing his face; Elvis asks him for his help but Giani refuses, leaving Elvis to carry Min into one of the cubicles. Giani claims to have seen Elvis kissing Polly. Elvis becomes enraged as Giani begins to preach to him. Giani asks Elvis to kill him, there is a tussle between them and Giani's turban falls off. Elvis launches himself again at the old man. Min comes out of the cubicle and tells Elvis to stop.

Min then delivers an impassioned speech criticising the superficiality of the elders in their community, and for the fact that appearances must be preserved. She expresses her contempt for the glitzy outward appearance of members of her faith as well as her dashed hopes for the future. Her anger is tempered by her belief that she is not, like the others, pretending and that she prays to see if God will help them all. Elvis responds by asking to take care of Min, but she tells him that all she does is look after other people. Gradually, however, the mood softens as Min expresses her love for Elvis. Elvis in turn asks her to leave with him, but Min says she cannot. Undeterred, Elvis says that he'll help Min learn about life outside the community. Min is cautious and explains that Elvis doesn't know anything about Min personally. Elvis says that he knows that Min dances, yet Min tells him she is sometimes violent. Together they begin to talk about renewal and change, and the fact that they can start again from this moment. Min dances and holds Elvis's hand, Elvis pulls her towards him and they embrace. The intimacy is broken by a violent scream offstage, as well as the sound of falling cutlery. Elvis rushes to see what has happened but is stopped by Teetee. Balbir enters, dazed, and displays her hands which are covered in blood. Balbir takes Min's head in her hands, and the mother and daughter whisper praises to God. Min draws away and reaches out to touch Elvis as the lights fade and the play comes to an end.

MODERN INTERPRETATION

The notion of 'culture', as we have seen, is a complex one. Clearly, the focus of *Behzti* is on the culture of the contemporary Sikh community, but its themes (silence in the face of abuse, the pressure to conform to social 'norms') are of course applicable in other cultural contexts. If we survey the plays that we have explored so far, we can see some parallels between the narratives in terms of culture (in the sense of the environment and in terms of a system of values). There is the repression of feelings and guilt that we can witness in *Cloud 9*, *Little Eyolf*, *All My Sons* and *Journey's End* and the claustrophobia and menace of *The Caretaker*.

Behzti became known in some quarters as 'That Sikh Play', which is reductive as it effectively marginalises this powerful play and renders it culturally specific. The play has universal relevance in its portrayal of a community that is bound by a particular belief system, but undermined when individuals exploit this system. The play carefully exposes how wrongdoing can be facilitated when individuals feel they cannot speak out for fear of reprisals from senior members of the community.

Silence is an important catalyst for the narrative of *Behtzi*. The playwright herself effectively broke the silence of the issue of sexual abuse in the Sikh community. Yet the play itself is crafted to create tension through implication. Balbir's oblique references to Mr Sandhu's 'list' generate an ominous atmosphere, while Min herself effectively stays silent rather than standing up to her bad-tempered mother. There is also the persuasive sense in the play of the 'old ways' that must not be challenged or addressed.

In *The Caretaker* we observed that Aston was betrayed by his social circle for 'saying things' (we infer Aston's comments were found 'abnormal' by his peers). Aston is sectioned because he is vocal and defies the social norms. We cannot of course know specifically how Aston has behaved, but the end result is that the man has been broken psychologically and is effectively 'silenced' and consequently exploited and violated by Davies in a similar way to how Mr Sandhu exploits Min's quiet but firm faith.

CLINICAL CONTEXTS

Culture consists of the beliefs, values and behaviours that exist among groups in society.[5] Through our culture we define who we are, to what extent we share values and how we contribute to our society. Cultural sensitivity refers to the doctor's understanding of how culture may impact on a patient's choices and the doctor's ability to respect differences.[5] Koffman and Crawley suggest that our goal while working clinically should be to identify 'differences that make a difference' among patients.[6] Culture is sometimes seen as a narrow concept, a checklist of behaviours and rituals, which, although important, risks encouraging generalisations about individuals as a result of their cultural background. This risks leading to prejudice and stereotyping. Culture is more appropriately viewed as a wider dynamic concept which changes as a result of interactions with others. We notice in *Behzti* how a stifling, subverted notion of Sikhism both disempowers the characters (such as Min's accusations of rape being disbelieved by those who should love her the most) but is also perpetuated by the dishonesty – seen in Polly and Teetee's theft of shoes from the Gurdwara.

Although much of the literature in this area focuses on culture with reference to patients and their families in ethnic minority groups, doctors and other healthcare professionals share a *medical culture* in addition to any issues of their own ethnicity and cultural background. Doctors have a medical language and use jargon and acronyms to describe the symptoms, signs and illnesses they encounter in their practice. Furthermore, within the medical culture there is a shared culture in palliative care evidenced by terms such as 'hospice movement'. Doctors need to be aware of their own culture and how this affects their interaction with patients. This becomes even more complex when one considers the cultural impact on medical practice when the doctor comes from a minority ethnic group or holds religious convictions which differ from those of the patient. There may be external pressures which makes providing culturally appropriate care more challenging, such as demands from an increase in the ageing population and working with shrinking resources. If we take a broad view of culture, then cross-cultural interactions become much more complex than exercises in interpreting the other's language or behaviours but develop into true dialogues which carry the potential for change in both parties. In this dynamic process of exchange both parties gain new insights; in addition to improved communication there is a space for more significant attitudinal changes such as sensitivity or humility that are the basis of patient-centred care.[6]

It is puzzling that members of ethnic minorities do not access specialist palliative care services to any great extent.[7] If we are to improve access to end-of-life care there must be a commitment to deliver culturally appropriate care. Any prescriptive approach to multiculturalism risks stereotyping individuals so doctors need to understand the individual's belief system and to strive to minimise inequalities in the power relations between doctor and patient. Culturally appropriate care is based on mutual trust and respect for each other's nationality, culture, age, gender and religious beliefs.[8]

Behzti provides striking insights into Sikh culture which resonates with issues facing ethnic minorities in end-of-life care. Drama is one way in which we can explore 'the other' and increase our understanding of the patient's social and cultural background.[9] Western culture embodies certain ideas about self-hood, patienthood, illness and care which differ from the beliefs and views of non-Western patients and doctors.[10] One of the central questions addressed in our book is 'How can I see the world through the patient's eyes?' Part of the response to this question is to try to understand social and cultural differences. Sometimes difference is valued as simple diversity, but more often it is identified as being a negative deviation from the norms of the dominant group.[11] 'Otherness' is an extreme version of this where the dominant group defines itself in opposition to the marginalised group.[11]

In *Behzti*, this can be observed by Mr Sandhu's cruel rejection of Biloo's services for the extension to the Gurdwara, stating his belief that the job is not suitable for Indians and in this respect undermines his own cultural context.

'Othering' can reinforce situations of domination and subordination with the risk that characteristics may be projected onto a marginalised group and assumptions made which lead to stereotyping. We need to be cautious that 'othering' may lead to a lack of understanding of a particular individual by labelling anything non-compliant with normative medical practice as 'culture'.[11] Rather than applying simple labels we should explore what difference means. Instead of fixing existing power relationships between doctors and their patients, with cultural sensitivity we can become closer to our patients.[11]

IDENTITY

As well as culture, identity can be based on a host of categories: race, ethnicity, citizenship, gender, religion, politics, sexual orientation and social class being some examples.[6] Race only embodies the minor differences which exist between populations reflecting external characteristics such as facial features and colour, so should not be regarded as a significant determinant of identity, as we have observed in *Cloud 9*.

Ethnicity is a way of grouping people on the basis of historical or territorial identity or by shared cultural traditions maintained through generations.[6] Ethnicity may be defined by language; for example, Hispanic people in America or by a shared ancestry such as African Americans. To complicate matters people alter their ethnic group with time, and there is evidence that they have multiple identities which are expressed differently as circumstances change.[6] This is important for clinicians to remember when they interpret a patient's story with regard to culture, race and ethnicity. It is vital to explore the patient's particular needs, beliefs and choices without preconceptions and understand that patients may face particular cultural pressures that may well be outside the practitioner's own experience.

CULTURAL RELATIVISM

Cultural relativism (multiculturalism) is defined as 'a social–intellectual movement that promotes the value of diversity as a core principle and insists that all cultural groups be treated with respect as equals'.[12] To ensure equitable access to palliative care services we need to address any relevant differences between groups. This is not to equate cultural relativism with ethical relativism; that is, respect for diversity does not mean accepting a violation of another's human rights. In end-of-life care there are a number of important areas where cultural differences have a particular impact on the effectiveness of care.

Patients and their families may have different preferences in their wish to receive honest information about a life-threatening disease and the extent to which they wish to be involved in decision making. For example, Annie, a young Chinese student who has advanced bowel cancer, is unwilling for doctors to discuss her diagnosis either with her or to mention the fact she is ill to her parents in China since cancer is considered shameful in her culture. We observe in *Behtzi* how notions of 'shame' and 'dishonour' can be difficult to understand (or indeed condone). Yet as many commentators have asserted, this is not a play that attacks Sikhism per se, but highlights the tensions and cruelty when a belief system is exploited.

Ari is a Muslim man dying of a sarcoma which is causing him great pain. Ari asked for opioids to relieve his pain, but his family insist that he should not receive painkillers, believing that his suffering was a test of faith.[6]

In Western cultures and particularly in the United States, autonomy is given the highest priority of the ethical principles since these cultures value individualism. In Eastern society and Africa, on the other hand, beneficence is more valued so a family and community approach is more of a priority. Indeed individuals might fear being marginalised from their family and community group and would tend to seek their involvement in decisions about their care.

Thus the locus of decision making in Western cultures is largely the patient, whereas in other cultures in Asia it is more often the family. The Western approach of an internal locus of control places the individual as determining their own fate whereas the non-Western approach may be more fatalistic, believing that events are predetermined by fate or the gods.

Advanced care planning is thus an activity which many people in the West are comfortable with as they wish control over the manner of their death. Indeed some people wish to control not only the manner of their dying but the timing of it so are demanding euthanasia to be legalised. It is interesting that there is no such public demand for euthanasia from Eastern countries.

Some patients may not trust doctors as a result of abuse of minority groups in the past. An instance would be the legacy of the notorious Tuskegee syphilis experiment on African Americans which has resulted in many African Americans being suspicious of their doctor's motives and so demanding life-prolonging treatments at the end of life even when they are futile.[13] More recently, in Pakistan, the murder by the Taliban of healthcare workers administering polio vaccine was justified by the killers who claimed the medical staff were part of a conspiracy on behalf of the West who were experimenting on or sterilising the young patients.

To address cultural issues the doctor must explore cultural beliefs, address issues of spirituality and religion and build trust with the patient and their family. Cultural differences between groups are a helpful guide to a patient's beliefs, but they are not protocols for care. We have seen in the controversy spawned by *Behzti*'s premiere in Birmingham how easily a theatrical exploration of particular practices can be construed a generalised assault on an entire culture. Cultural sensitivity depends on a creative use of silence and forces the doctor to listen. Different cultures may require different models of explaining illness. In the West there is a biomedical approach, but in other cultures the balance between health and illness is perceived differently. In some Hindu cultures, for example, a present cancer may be seen as a punishment for sins in an earlier life.

Doctors should not make assumptions about a patient from a particular minority group but listen to their individual needs. Examples of how such conversations may be facilitated include questions such as:

- What do you think has caused your illness?
- What worries you most about your illness?
- Are you the kind of person who wants to know all the information about your illness?
- Do you prefer to leave decisions to the doctor?
- Do you prefer to make decisions or would you like your family to decide?
- Would you like to be present when I speak with your family?
- Is there anything in your culture that would be helpful for us to know?
- Are there any particular beliefs or practices you feel we should know about?
- What are your concerns about death and dying?
- Are there any particular types of medical intervention you would like to forego?
- Are there any practices around death that we should know about?

Good end-of-life care strives to meet the needs of the individual. In *Behzti*, it is never clear whether Min's caring for Balbir is simply through a sense of filial duty or a commitment that is determined by her cultural identity. The playwright ostensibly suggests it is both, but then adds extra complexity to this relationship in Min's physical abuse of Balbir. These interactions are challenging and remind us that cultural and familial identity are often inextricably intertwined. Mr Sandhu's weary remark might strike a chord with families from a range of cultural backgrounds:

> SANDHU: Whatever things look like, there is always another story, always the truth underneath the show. After a while we get used to the disappointment. We don't even have to live with it because we pass our failures onto our children, like you [Min]. And everything becomes your problem.

Although we have emphasised that cultural sensitivity is much more than a checklist, there may be important rituals around dying and immediately after death which doctors need to be aware about. Palliative care and hospice care should be offered as an addition to the care provided by the family, not an alternative. By paying proper attention to the patient's views the doctor can listen to their cultural preferences. As we discussed in an earlier example, the patient may not wish to be informed directly of a life-threatening diagnosis but want their family to know. The reasons for non-disclosure should be explored: is it because it is in some way disrespectful or might it provoke depression? Is the concern that it will eliminate hope or even that talking about death and dying will bring about earlier death?

In open communication with members of ethnic minorities doctors may have to rely on translators who may have differing views from the patient and so unwittingly complicate the communication. 'Lost in translation' has become a cliché, but the phrase resonates with experience in a clinical context.

Communication difficulties may arise when there is reliance on the patient's relatives acting as interpreters on their behalf. The family interpreter may filter important information or represent their own view as that of either the doctor or the patient. Using friends or untrained interpreters also raises problems in maintaining confidentiality. Although *Behtzi*'s writer provides a glossary of Sikh terms at the end of the published play, much of the Sikh language in performance might well bewilder non-Sikh audience members, who, like Elvis, may feel alienated by this terminology. This is echoed in the Giani Jaswant's enigmatic meditations and the contrast between the modern pop CDs and the ceremonial chanting in the Gurdwara. Yet this multifaceted, fragmented use of language is an essential part of the play's power: what *do* these terms mean today? How have they become embedded in a culture? What role does ancient cultural tradition and language play in the rich, but often awkward, plurality of 21st-century Britain?

PROFESSIONAL CULTURES

Hall describes how each healthcare profession has a different culture which includes values, beliefs, attitudes, customs and behaviours.[14] These differing cultures have evolved over time and also reflect social class and gender issues. Education of students in differing disciplines reinforces these values in the jargon and attitudes of each profession.[14] Increasing specialisation has led to even further immersion of learners into the culture of their own professional group. These separate professional cultures may then hinder effective teamwork.[14] Healthcare professions have struggled to define their boundaries; nursing may be perceived to challenge the authority and boundaries of medicine. It is not just in their education but in socialisation processes which also serve to cement the professionals' particular view.[12] Doctors, for instance, traditionally learn in a competitive environment whereas nurses learn early in their career to work as a team. Medical students may not be exposed to the humanities so further solidifying biomedical attitudes. A challenge for interprofessional team-working is for team members to understand each other's background and culture. Palliative care has developed team-working, and values listening to others' stories. Role blurring in palliative care teams is used as a positive force since it fosters creative approaches to problem solving. However, when tired and stressed, healthcare professionals can withdraw into their silos. It is sad when professionals maintain their boundaries at the expense of the patient's welfare. A clinical example of such inappropriate behaviour follows.

Jill, a district nurse, and Robert, a GP, felt they knew how to manage a patient dying of lung cancer at home. Despite having difficulties in relieving the patient's breathlessness, they were reluctant to call a specialist palliative care nurse for advice for fear of being criticised for their management of the patient. Similarly, in *Behtzi* there is discord over the signing of Elvis's 'sheet' for his care of Balbir. What *is* his role? Min exposes this tension in her angry critique of Elvis's naivety and essentially his 'otherness':

> MIN (shouts): You have no right to address me. You're not even anything to do with me, you're here for her and look . . . you're prancing around, in this religious area, saying things. Things that don't concern me. You're flipping well home care, right, and that's all! Get out of my way.

Yet culture provides a way of communicating with those around us; membership of different cultures allows us to gain insight. Culture is a voice we communicate with, but it also is the eyes and ears through which we receive communication: silent treatment.[11]

Isaiah Berlin in 'Two Concepts of Liberty' says: 'When I am among my own people they understand me, as I understand them; and this understanding creates within me a sense of being somebody in the world.'[15]

This insight emphasises the relational aspect of autonomy; I am a person through other people. This patient-centred view can be contrasted with 'I think therefore I am' which takes a narrow self-orientated view of autonomy. Sharing of space, of community, refers not simply to physical space but the psychological connection of living with others. Ideas of culture are of cultivating a relationship with others in a community. The implication for clinicians is that they must be prepared to learn from patients. To fail to try to understand people's suffering within the cultural terms in which they experience their distress is to fail to respect their dignity. Palliative care relies on attention to detail and nowhere is this more important than in understanding cultural differences and avoiding stereotyping. A patient's sense of security depends not just on tolerance of difference or diversity but on respect, a more powerful virtue than simply tolerance. Insecurities about one's own cultural identity can nurture prejudice. The busy environment of clinical care and the pressure to make quick clinical decisions are factors which can, unfortunately, lead healthcare professionals to ignore cultural complexity and to opt for simplifying the situation by stereotyping.

MODELS OF CONNECTION

Model of connecting with 'the other'

Phillips *et al.* describe how kindness can connect the self and the other.[19] In the 17th century, before the Enlightenment, kindness was viewed as a bridge between the Self and the Other which acted to promote goodwill and to maintain social solidarity. Kindness here is seen as patronage; the 'self' is isolated from the 'other'.

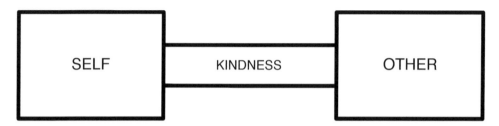

FIGURE 9.1 Pre-modern model: 'The Bridge'

An alternative post-modern model: 'connection'

Here the 'self' is integral with the 'other' and each is mutually dependent on the other. This reflects the reality of our shared vulnerability and sees kindness as a way of maintaining close relations. As Ralph Waldo Emerson said, 'It is one of the beautiful compensations of life that no man can sincerely try to help another without helping himself.'[20]

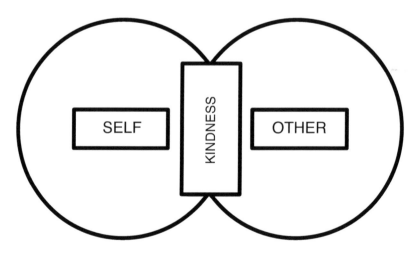

FIGURE 9.2 Post-modern model: 'Connection'

CONCLUSION

Cross-cultural ethical dilemmas should be seen as relational problems. In coming to the optimal solution the goal of all involved should be to seek understanding and consensus not blame the 'other' for being wrong.[6] Cultural, religious and ethnic groups should be treated as equals while at the same time any practices which threaten fundamental human rights should not be tolerated. There is good evidence that inequalities exist with respect to race, ethnicity and access to specialist palliative care.[7,16] Koffman and Crawley examine the reasons for Black and ethnic minority exclusion from end-of-life care in both the USA and UK.[6] They describe a number of factors including social and economic deprivation, poor knowledge of specialist palliative care services, bias in provider services, differing attitudes to palliative care, dissatisfaction with services and cultural mistrust. It may be that although there is not conscious discrimination, which we all reject, there may be more subtle underlying unconscious attitudes which influence our behaviour when under pressure.[6]

Koffman and Crawley look at the following domains for providing palliative care for culturally diverse populations.[6]

Pain

The way in which pain and other symptoms are experienced, understood and expressed by patients may be affected by their culture and many other factors. For example, some African Caribbean patients in the UK perceive pain as a test of religious faith or as divine punishment.[16]

Psychosocial and spiritual

Caring for family members is an important duty for many ethnic minority communities. In Hindu families' concepts of karma, which emphasise the future, consequences of neglecting sacred duties may impose burdens on the family. They may feel they have to cope with their dying relative at home even when this is no longer practical. There may be an underlying assumption that ethnic minority patients have no spiritual problems because they have their own beliefs and they look after each other.[6] This is another example of averting attention from the difficult area of spiritual care, a form of collusion which leaves the patient unsupported and excluded. Experience of an illness has a meaning for the individual patient who must remain in the foreground of care. The expression of this meaning for the individual patient is influenced by many factors including their culture which can be seen as the background. The challenge for those caring for the patient is to keep both in focus. We need to decipher how much of the patient's distress is an expression of their cultural background and strive to understand the patient's problem in the terms that the patient experiences them.[18]

Culture is not a problem to be overcome, or something that clouds the essential truth, but is rather an integral part of the patient's story. Different cultures create different experiences, expression and consequences of suffering and those responding to this suffering should be prepared to see the world through the individual patient's eyes. We should be prepared to follow the patient's agenda and to explore how patients use their culture as a medium of communication through which to express their suffering. The patient is not the object of treatment but the subject of concern. This can be affirmed by listening to their subjective experience and interpretation of their problem. Healthcare professionals need to understand how people comprehend their illness and to determine what sort of help they need.

REFERENCES

1 *Daily Telegraph* editorial. Available online at: www.asiansinmedia.org/news/article. php/radio/759 (accessed 16 January 2013).

2 Singh M. Theatre stormed in Sikh protest. BBC news. Available online at: http://news. bbc.co.uk/1/hi/england/west_midlands/4107437.stm (accessed 16 January 2013).

3 Wilde Y. Talk with Sikhs 'backfired' on theatre. *The Guardian*. Available online at: www.guardian.co.uk/uk/2004/dec/29/arts.religion (accessed 16 January 2013).

4 Sharp R. Behzti is no longer taboo. Available online at: www.robertsharp. co.uk/2010/05/06/behzti-is-no-longer-taboo/ (accessed 16 January 2013).

5 Clark D. Cultural considerations in planning palliative and end of life care. *Palliat Med*. 2012; **26**: 195–6.

6 Koffman J, Crawley L. Ethnic and cultural aspects of palliative medicine. In: Hanks G, Christakis N, Cherny N *et al*, editors. *The Oxford Textbook of Palliative Medicine*. 4th ed. Oxford: Oxford University Press; 2010.

7 Firth S. *Wider Horizons: care of the dying in a multi-cultural society*. London: National Council for Hospices and Specialist Palliative Care Services; 2001.

8 Clarke K, Phillips J. End of life care: the importance of culture and ethnicity. *Aust Fam Physician*. 2012; **39**:21.

9 Matharu KS, Howell J, Fitzgerald FT. Fearlessly exploring the other: the role of drama in medical training. *Med Humanities*, 2010; **36**: 58–9.

10 Hooker C, Noonan E. Medical humanities as expressive of Western culture. *Med Humanit*. 2011; **37**: 79–84.

11 MacLachlan M. *Culture and Health*. Chichester: John Wiley and Sons; 2006.

12 Macklin R. Ethical relativism in a multicultural society. *Kennedy Inst Ethics J*. 1998; **8**: 1–22.

13 Tuskegee Syphilis Study. Available online at: www.sciencemuseum.org.uk/brought tolife/techniques/tuskegee.aspx (accessed 7 January 2013).

14 Hall P. Interprofessional teamwork: professional cultures as barriers. *J Interprof Care*. 2005; **1**: 188–96.

15 Berlin I. Two concepts of liberty. In: Berlin I. *Four Essays on Liberty*. Oxford: Oxford University Press; 1969.

16 Olivere D. Culture and ethnicity. *Eur J Palliat Care*. 1999; **6**: 53–6.

17 Koffman J, Morgan M, Edmonds P *et al*. Cultural meanings of pain: a qualitative study of Black Caribbean and White British patients with advanced cancer. *Palliat Med*. 2008; **22**: 349–59.

18 Ward C, Bochner S *et al*. *The Psychology of Culture Shock*. London: Routledge; 2001.

19 Phillips A, Taylor B. *On Kindness*. London: Penguin Books; 2009.

20 Emerson RW. *Selected Writings of Ralph Waldo Emerson*. New York: Penguin Putnam; 2011.

CHAPTER 10

Cooperation: drama and healthcare education

INTRODUCTION

Although drama has not been used in medical education to the same extent as other forms of the arts and humanities, Kohn believes there is a place for the study of theatre in medical education. He presents convincing arguments for bringing performance, actors and theatre educators into medical education.[1] Role play, a form of drama, is widely used in communication skills training for medical students.[2] Play reading and street theatre have also been used in medical training abroad to develop empathy.[3,4] Macneill argues the humanities should take a more active role in medical education by challenging the assumptions of the biomedical model.[5] He suggests that recent work in the arts and humanities, which may initially be difficult to understand, may provoke open discussion and critical reflection among medical students and healthcare professionals and so enhance their personal development.[5]

We describe 'Performance and Palliative Care: A Drama Module for Medical Students', a two-week Student Selected Component (SSC) module developed in Dundee Medical School.[6] Students examined ways in which drama and theatre can be used in medical practice through interrogating concepts such as performance, empathy, uncertainty and ethics. Practical drama workshops using improvisation and games-playing were combined with student-led discussion groups and tutorials on end-of-life care. Lessons learned from the drama sessions were related to clinical scenarios so enabling students to enhance their understanding of doctor–patient communication in difficult situations. The play studied was *The Caretaker* by Harold Pinter, which students read before the beginning of the module.[7] *The Caretaker* was chosen as it illustrates a number of themes which are central to end-of-life care: silence, power, care, uncertainty and communication[8] (*see* Chapter 2).

The students wrote a reflective portfolio and performed a short play at the end of the module based on their learning outcomes.

The module aimed to provide students with the opportunity to develop a creative approach to problem solving and to gain a better understanding of the patient's experience. It was hoped that they would have greater confidence in dealing with uncertainty and would improve their team-working skills. Students were encouraged to take risks, to express their views and to engage with the content and opportunities offered in this innovative module. The relaxed, non-judgemental atmosphere of the workshop helped the students to feel free to express their views.

Drama games were a way for students on the SSC to investigate and 'tap into' perspectives not covered in more conventional learning methods.[9] They also acted as a device to decrease anxiety about 'getting things right', encouraging students to experiment. The students did not know each other before coming to the course so these games acted as 'icebreakers' and helped build a relaxed learning environment from the outset.

The students worked in trios, drawing an outline around one group member on paper and then drawing in the attributes of the 'good' doctor. The participants emphasised differing virtues and realised that while we share notions of a 'bad' doctor, it is harder to define the 'good' doctor. They all emphasised the importance of a listening ear and broad shoulders!

Students were ambivalent about the use of reflection; many had experiences of reflection as a tick-box exercise which they had not found a helpful learning experience. The students were reassured that since an aim of this module was to encourage creativity they should not feel constrained, but use the reflection in a way that was meaningful for them. This course was not about intellectual drama criticism. Rather we wanted to ensure that we encouraged students to feel free to express their feelings and to know that their opinions were valid and helpful in informing the discussions. Once we had explained that reflection could be an individual or group activity, in written or spoken form, students felt more enthusiastic. They were also given time each day during the course to make notes for their reflection.

Similarly, students were reassured that the end of course performance could take different forms. They agreed that they would split into three trios and each trio would write a 15-minute play which they would perform and which focused on a module theme. They were given time and advice during rehearsal to prepare for this assessment.

In exploring the use of silence we looked at situations where it was appropriate to wait, to say nothing as well as identifying how silence could damage effective communication. Pauses were created in the module to allow time for individual and group reflection and for problem solving. Giving space allowed every student to contribute during each session of the module. Conversations around power increased the students' awareness of staging, of how to set up the room like a performance. They explored how they felt in relation to one another in experiencing power.

The students discussed how words in a medical context may have a different – or opposite – meaning to layperson. For example, the notion of the 'progression' of cancer might mistakenly be seen as positive to a patient. The group explored some difficult communication issues which might arise in terminal care. These included place of care, withdrawal of treatments, feeling a burden, and loss of dignity. Chochinov's model of ABCD of Dignity Care was used to give the students a practical framework for enhancing patient dignity[10] (*see* Chapter 7).

The students investigated how they might respond to a patient's plea: 'Help me to die.' After discussing the practical communication issues behind this question we turned to debate the ethics of euthanasia and assisted suicide. It has become a hot topic again with the prospect of renewed interest in legislation in Scotland.[11] The students were asked to reflect on their views and then to position themselves across the room according to how strongly they agreed or disagreed with the legalisation of euthanasia. The group split almost in half so they were then asked to sit at opposite ends and to debate the issue. Everyone felt confident to express a view and those students who felt really strongly listened respectfully to those with a different view. We concluded that this was a topic in which people were polarised in their view, but we all shared an urge to reduce suffering.

An early discussion of the term 'care' was enlightening and a helpful entry point to this complex notion both in the palliative context and in Pinter's play. Early conversations with the group elicited phrases such as 'providing comfort', 'alleviating pain' and 'reassurance'. There was also some deliberation on the negative connotations of the phrase 'taken into care'; the question was also raised that while a doctor clearly should 'care' *for* her patients (that is, provide treatment), should she actually 'care' *about* them (that is, concern herself over the ultimate outcome of their illness)?

Different dimensions of 'care' (responsibility, nurture, treatment and anxiety) are the cornerstones of the palliative care experience. The planning and delivery of the module showed care in listening to the students' concerns. The group cared when a student was late or absent from a session. They appreciated the importance of attention to detail and of putting the other person first. Their care for each other was demonstrated in their mutual support during the performances at the end of the module.

The students were introduced to the various types of roles people may play in a caring team. The technique of a group sculpt, a silent form of role play, was used to look at the various people involved with the care of a patient dying of cancer at home.[2] We used the story of a young mother dying from lung cancer and the group identified the key people involved in her care at home. Each student was given a role. The 'patient' sat in the centre of the room and then we positioned the other students, in role, depending on how close or important they were to her. The students then stood in these positions and were given a chance to say how they felt about where they had been placed. They then had an opportunity to move to a position where they felt more comfortable. Sculpting can be a powerful way of exploring team dynamics and relationships.

Medical students and doctors are not good at taking care of themselves. Doctors have high rates of alcohol abuse, broken marriages and stress.[12] The group split into pairs and identified what caused them stress: workload, responsibility, fear of not knowing what to do, a lack of confidence and the difficulty of maintaining a work/life balance emerged as prominent themes.

We then had a group discussion on ways of reducing stress. An important learning point was that it is part of a doctor's professional duty to look after their own health, and to seek help with stress is the proper professional response.

Uncertainty is a problematic notion for medical students (in the same way, as below, unanswered questions can be frustrating), but uncertainty lies at the heart of both the work of Pinter and in a clinical context. Pinter writes that 'a thing may not necessarily be true or false – it may both be true *and* false': in the context of his plays one can see evidence of this in the fragile, subjective memories of different characters attempting to ascertain what happened in the past.[13] A deconstruction of some of the uncertainties within Pinter's work may shed light on ambiguities in the end-of-life care environment. For instance, the group explored the difficulties in discussing prognosis with patients and their families.

A group role play was used to explore the response to a patient's question: 'How long have I got?' Although some members of the group maintained that they would like a doctor to be quite direct, the group came to appreciate the importance of a more gradual approach which explored the patient's under-standing before imparting a prognosis. They took away the learning point 'Ask then tell' and appreciated the difficulty of giving a prognosis.

Unanswered questions are fundamental to Pinter's art: from mysterious interrogations in the early plays to philosophical 'questioning' of one's exist-ence and the reliability of memory in later works. The majority of Pinter's questions (posed by the characters, or, indeed, posed by the play to the audi-ence) remain unanswered. Pinter talks about his writing process in terms of 'picking up clues' from his characters: he sees them as organic beings that will emerge as he develops the play. For medical students and doctors, questions are clearly at the heart of taking a case history, and the 'clues' they must pick up may be as opaque or apparently inconsistent as any of Pinter's narratives or characters.

Pinter's plays can also provide an insight into *how* questions are asked. In his first play *The Birthday Party*, the reclusive character Stanley is famously sub-jected to a surreal interrogation where questions are illogical, contradictory and impossible to answer.[14] Davies, in *The Caretaker*, is mercilessly probed about his shadowy past by his tormentor, Mick. In turn, Aston and Davies have a muted conversation about the possible implications of a woman's apparently sugges-tive 'question' in a café. In this SSC we were keen to consider the implications of particular questioning strategies, and the psychological implications of phrasing questions in a particular way.

We used the story of a young mother with a baby who is constantly going to her GP with worries about her daughter's health. The story was read and discussed. The students listed all the characters who might be involved in the story. Each student took a character and spent time thinking about the story from that perspective. Each person then told the story from their perspective.

The students appreciated that by listening to each other's stories and subsequently reflecting on them in the group, a more complex picture emerges. They became more aware of the limitations of their own perspective and the need to listen to others to gain a wider understanding of the patient's situation.

PERFORMANCE

There were three student performances on the last day of the module. The first explored issues of power in the consultation by using the patient's notes in the same way as Pinter used Davies' bag in *The Caretaker*. The second explored silence and emotions in end-of-life care. This performance ended with a student, playing the dying patient's husband, singing to the group.

The third play looked at doctor–patient communication by illustrating a 'bad' doctor then a 'good' doctor. Each performance was filmed so that the students would have a record of their work for their portfolios. It was gratifying to see how much effort the students put into scripting each play and to see students who had expressed reservations about role play, only a fortnight earlier, taking part in the short plays with sensitivity and enthusiasm. After each play the actors received feedback on their performance from their peers and from the tutors.

The group had a discussion on performance anxiety: where certain individuals are prone to exaggerated, often incapacitating anxiety in situations of public exposure or competitive scrutiny. Much of the work on this topic has been on musicians and actors, but this type of anxiety is common among medical students on ward rounds, and clinical exams such as OSCEs. We discussed the features of performance anxiety and identified perfectionist personalities as being particularly at risk. It was beyond the scope of this module to explore all the approaches to deal with this, but students had a brief description of the use of mindfulness meditation in dealing with anxiety.[15]

REFLECTIVE ESSAYS

A few extracts from the students' reflections are included by way of illustration:

> On entering the room to start the role play I tried to block my mind from what I was about to do – 'perform' in front of a group of people I had only known for one week. In the end everything went really well and I realised that it was such a small thing to worry about. I clearly make a big deal out of scenarios that I think are daunting when others around me are not judging me to the extent I believe they are.
>
> During the module I have learnt a lot about myself as a person and what makes a good doctor as a result of this I have set myself targets. One of which is to talk less and let the patient speak more, another is to remain unbiased in ethical dilemmas.
>
> I thought about how Morag's [the patient's] perspective would change as her life came closer to its end. Sometimes as a doctor it could be easy to focus completely on the illness and how the illness affects their life and forget about how not only her illness affects those around her but how the attitudes and connections of those around her can affect her both mentally and physically.
>
> The play opened my eyes to these issues and many more. It won me over from my initial scepticism and made me realise that in the future when deciding on a seemingly minor point like chair positioning, time does need to be spent to ensure that it's in the best possible place for the situation.

OUTCOMES AND EVALUATION

The students all felt that they had achieved the learning outcomes for the module.

> Its probably the most I have learned about reflection throughout my time at medical school. I thought the learning outcomes were covered really well.

It has been good to dedicate time to communication skills and ethics in a new and enjoyable way.

Great course, very useful and I believe I have learned skills and had experiences which will remain with me throughout my medical career.

DISCUSSION

In formulating this interdisciplinary module, there was an initial tension in considering how the text should be presented to the medical students and, crucially, if there needed to be a different approach from teaching students of drama. In terms of a Drama Studies module, the process would usually be for the students to have a preliminary discussion of the text ('table work') which might be supplemented by looking at broad critical discourses surrounding Pinter's work (such as Martin Esslin's seminal book *The Theatre of the Absurd* (1961) and Michael Billington's authoritative biography *The Life and Work of Harold Pinter* (1996).[16,17] This would then be followed by initial practical workshops to explore particular themes – through improvisation and games – in order to gain an understanding of the play as a whole.

What became clear from the first meetings with the students was that there was some anxiety around the study of *The Caretaker*, particularly in terms of 'getting' the play or seeing its relevance to their work as young doctors. Part of this anxiety appeared to stem from the prospect of assessment, particularly in terms of grading. Further, the open-ended nature of Pinter's play was seen, understandably, as intimidating in terms of finding 'answers'. Whereas we might be accustomed to locate a particular ideology or 'message' from a play, Pinter has warned against writing from a 'moral principle' and has said, 'I can sum up none of my plays. All I can say is: that is what happened. That is what they said. That is what they did.'[13] Part of the initial discussion, therefore, was geared towards finding the open nature of the text as an opportunity rather than a threat.

It can be challenging for medical students to consider practice which can be uncertain and complex to negotiate. It is useful to use other modes of learning to introduce new approaches offered by drama strategies which can lead to new knowledge generation, and provide alternatives ways of approaching problems.[18] Brunt refers to the need for healthcare professionals to develop critical thinking skills to address increasingly complex problems.[18] She states that critical thinking is necessary to create practitioners who are independent in their thinking, who can respond adequately to the needs of patients. As well as being logical, critical and pragmatic, critical thinking is helpfully augmented by such qualities as creativity, imagination, insight and intuition.[19]

The students were engaged with the issues and found the fresh approach of drama teachers challenged the biomedical view of medicine. Students who initially expressed reservations about the use of reflection or role play and had low confidence levels flourished during the course. After two weeks they wrote and presented performances which provided evidence of significant learning and insight in relation to issues of care, power, silence and uncertainty as expressed by Harold Pinter's *The Caretaker*.

It is important to embed the lessons from drama into clinical practice. We focused on palliative care and, in particular, end-of-life care as this is something which touches the practice of every doctor. Despite having no previous exposure to palliative care training, the students enjoyed the difficult communication scenarios and approached the ethical debate in a structured and respectful way. Clinical care depends on teamwork and the forging of a learning team in two weeks among students who did not know each other before this module was another positive outcome.

Narratives have been used to trigger reflection in another SSC in Dundee.[20] Hammer *et al.* describe a way of using storytelling and theatre to improve case presentation skills.[21] However, the model we used was that of McDrury and Alterio developed in New Zealand which uses story construction and reconstruction in a group setting to foster deep learning.[22]

The students' enthusiasm and engagement with the course, their performances, storytelling and writing reflections showed a wish to grasp the complexities of end-of-life care. This has convinced us that this form of short theatre workshop can play a useful part in medical students' professional development particularly with regard to confidence, self-awareness, ethical thinking and communication skills. The workshop also was useful in enhancing the students' capacity for reflection and insight.

REFERENCES

1 Kohn M. Performing medicine: the role of theatre in medical education. *Med Humanit.* 2011; **37**: 3–4.

2 Jeffrey D, editor. *Teaching Palliative Care: a practical guide.* Oxford: Radcliffe Medical Press; 2002.

3 Matharu KS, Howell J, Fitzgerald FT. Fearlessly exploring the other: the role of drama in medical training. *Med Humanit.* 2010; **36**: 58–9.

4 Gupta S, Singh S. Confluence: understanding medical humanities through street theatre. *Med Humanit.* 2011; **37**: 127–8.

5 Macneill PU The arts and medicine: a challenging relationship. *Med Humanit.* 2011; **37**: 85–90.

6 Jeffrey EJ, Goddard J, Jeffrey D. Performance and Palliative Care: a drama module for medical students. *Med Humanit.* 2012; **38**: 110–14.

7 Pinter H. *The Caretaker.* London: Methuen; 1960.

8 Jeffrey EJ, Jeffrey D. I could never quite get it together: lessons for end-of-life care in Harold Pinter's *The Caretaker. Med Humanit.* 2012; **33**: 117–26.

9 Heathcote D, Bolton, G. *Drama for Learning: Dorothy Heathcote's mantle of the expert approach to education.* Portsmouth: Heinemann; 1996.

10 Chochinov H. Dignity and the essence of medicine: the A,B,C, and D of dignity conserving care. *BMJ.* 2007; **335**: 184–7.

11 Mcdonald M. Assisted Suicide (Scotland) Bill 2012. A Consultation Paper. Available online at: www.scottish.parliament.uk/S4_MembersBills/Final_version_as_lodged.pdf (accessed 9 February 2012).

12 McVeigh T. Alarm at rise of alcoholism in professions. *The Observer.* 13 November 2011. p. 19.

13 Pinter H. Writing for the theatre. In: *Plays One.* London: Faber; 1996.

14 Pinter H. *The Birthday Party.* In: *Plays One.* London: Faber; 1996.

15 Williams M, Penman D. *Mindfulness.* London: Piatkus; 2011.

16 Esslin M. *The Theatre of the Absurd.* London: Methuen; 1961.

17 Billington M. *The Life and Work of Harold Pinter.* London: Faber; 1996.

18 Brunt BA. Models, measurement, and strategies in developing critical-thinking skills. *J Contin Educ Nurs.* 2005; **36**(6): 255–62.

19 Walters K. *Re-thinking Reason: new perspectives in critical thinking.* Albany: State University of New York Press; 1994.

20 Law S. Using narratives to trigger reflection. *Clin Teach.* 2011; **8**: 147–50.

21 Hammer RR, Rian JD, Gregory JK *et al.,* Telling the patient's story: using theatre training to improve case presentation skills. *Med Humanit.* 2011; **37**: 18–22.

22 McDrury J, Alterio M. *Learning through Storytelling in Higher Education: using reflection and experience to improve learning.* London: Kogan Page; 2003.

CHAPTER 11

Combinations: virtue ethics
– the good doctor

'We are, all of us, pilgrims who struggle along different paths towards the same destination.'

Antoine de Saint-Exupéry

Science and technology have advanced doctors' abilities to extend life but possibly at the cost of putting patients at risk.[1] The pace of these scientific advances has overtaken the development of medical professionalism, creating a gulf between doctors and the society they serve.[2] Doctors are sometimes perceived to be limited in communication skills, empathy and openness, to be inaccessible and to be reluctant to admit to errors.[1] All societies need healers and to believe in their intrinsic virtue. However, in a market-driven world doctors' vocational drive has come under threat. The conflict between the profession's promotion of its own self-interests and its obligation to serve society was demonstrated in the recent strike by some doctors in the UK over their pension arrangements.[3] It is imperative that doctors and society understand the obligations associated with being a member of a profession. Doctors cannot function effectively as healers without the trust of patients and society.[2] New accountabilities manifest by revalidation and reaccreditation of doctors should help to restore trust between doctors, patients and society.

In *Tomorrow's Doctors* the General Medical Council describes the duties of a doctor; foremost of these is the duty 'to make the care of your patient your first concern'.[4] Putting patients first involves working with them and respecting them as individuals who have a right to be involved in decisions about their care. *Tomorrow's Doctors* gives guidance on the standards expected of a doctor in three categories: as a scientist, a practitioner and as a professional. It is this last category which we wish to explore in this final section of *Silent Treatment*. We explore the question: 'What is a good doctor?'

Standards of medical professionalism were described by Hippocrates who emphasised not only the duty of care to patients but the importance of respecting one's colleagues.[5]

There is no common definition of medical professionalism, although there is general agreement in appropriate attitudes, values and behaviours which are captured in the GMC's publication *Good Medical Practice*.[6] The core elements of a profession are possession of a specialised body of knowledge and a commitment to service.[7] This commitment to the patient means that professions are seen as altruistic and vocational. The commitment to altruism is the justification for the profession's autonomy to set standards of practice and for self-regulation to assure quality.

In considering the doctor as a professional the GMC refers to behaving according to ethical and legal principles laid out in *Good Medical Practice*: 'good doctors make the care of their patients their first concern: they are competent, keep their knowledge and skills up to date, establish and maintain good relationships with patients and colleagues, are honest and trustworthy, and act with integrity'.[6] They further stipulate that the doctor should be polite, considerate, trustworthy and honest, act with integrity, maintain confidentiality, respect patients' dignity and privacy and understand the importance of appropriate consent.[6] They are required to respect patients and colleagues regardless of cultural or social factors and to recognise the rights and equal value of all people.[6] Doctors have a duty to reflect on their practice, to continue their learning and to teach others. They should learn and work effectively with other healthcare professionals within a multiprofessional team.[2] These codes of behaviour describe some of the characteristics of a professional but somehow fail to capture the richness of what it is to be a good doctor. One reason for this may be that, generally, descriptions of medical professionalism are medically determined. The public seems to recognise doctors as professionals in a wider sense: by their good behaviour, high values and positive attitudes as clinicians, workers and citizens.[8]

Professionalism includes values which support the compassionate care of patients and is an integral part of medical practice and thus needs to be taught in medical schools.[9] All medical students to some degree struggle with the quantity and complexity of the factual knowledge that they are required to assimilate, they have anxieties about assessment and are encouraged to be competitive. Professional development is now an integral part of all medical schools, but the mechanisms for teaching it vary. Innovative teaching methods such as reflective portfolios, problem-based learning and using the arts and humanities have all been utilised in the hope of producing more 'rounded doctors'. Some research suggests that professional attitudes change little during medical training.[10] Good role models and mentoring are important in professional development as is the informal or hidden curriculum which includes social and cultural aspects that lie beyond the formal curriculum.[7,11]

Some unprofessional behaviours in medical students can predict likely future disciplinary action when they are doctors; severe irresponsibility, a diminished capacity for self-improvement and a failure to accept criticism were identified in one study.[13] Stern *et al.* found that a lack of humility or conscientiousness were warning signs for problem doctors.[14]

In this book we have attempted to draw parallels between the moral and ethical tensions in a range of plays and the challenges that a doctor may face in end-of-life care. These plays are striking not only in their representation of the human condition but in presenting problems, ambiguities and dilemmas. It is hoped that an understanding of the nature of these tensions will help doctors to develop empathy and compassion in difficult and uncertain circumstances.

These plays represent a complex series of interactions between relatives and surrogate or 'adopted' families. As audience members we must negotiate and interpret these for ourselves, but as doctors we must engage and interact with the complex 'families' of healthcare professionals, patients and their relatives. Just as the plays offer no easy answers, end-of-life care will often present complex situations where self-reflection and judgement are needed as well as good communication.

Phillips comments: 'If the best thing we do is look after each other, then the worst thing we do is pretend to look after each other when in fact we are doing something else.'[15] Phillips goes on to explore the notion of helping people in psychoanalytic terms. He describes psychoanalysis as a 'listening cure', a term which perhaps could be adopted for palliative care. It is in the listening relationship between the doctor and patient that each becomes aware of the other's needs. We have seen some of the ethical complexities which arise and are highlighted in end-of-life care. The whole process of caring for patients is fraught with moral dilemmas. Current ethical models which we have discussed, such as duty-based deontology or consequence-driven utilitarianism, do not seem sensitive to some of the most intricate dilemmas which arise at the end of life. Similarly, the four-principle approach which gives primacy to autonomy seems less helpful when dependency is inevitable at the end of life. Aristotle's virtue ethics provides a more useful basis to guide our actions at this time. Virtue ethics are more concerned with the development of the good doctor than with a principle-based analysis of the individual intervention or act.

Virtue is the concept of a good character. Annas points to two facets of virtue ethics: virtue as a practical skill and as a drive to aspire.[16] She suggests that just as we become more skilled at practical procedures by practice, so virtues require constant practice; we become generous by practising generosity. Thus virtues like kindness, compassion and empathy can be taught and this underlines the need for moral education from an early age.

A 'drive to aspire' is part of a doctor's professional development. Acquiring complex skills is more than a matter of copying experts. What the expert teaches is the need to understand the reasons why the doctor is doing a particular action and to learn from mistakes; that is, to become a reflective practitioner. In reflective practice the practitioner asks herself the Socratic question: 'How should I live?' The virtues are what enable the doctor to live well and to practice well.[17]

Virtue ethics seems a more appropriate model than a system of ethical rules. Virtue ethics takes account of emotions and imagination in developing empathy as a form of perceptual capacity.[5] The good doctor is one with practical wisdom (*phronesis*). 'Good' is hard to define, but it is not simply what is most easily measured.

Evidence-based medicine (EBM) uses the best available research-based evidence for making clinical decisions. Narrative-based medicine focuses on the patient's story and how the doctor and patient interact and interpret that story.

In this approach the world is viewed from the patient's perspective rather than from population-based evidence of EBM.[5]

EBM and narrative approaches are complementary and the good doctor is one who has the skill to use both with sensitivity by allowing for subjectivity, ambiguity and conflict in the individual patient. This focus on the individual patient lies at the heart of good decision making. The doctor must respond to the patient both intellectually and emotionally; to do this she needs to have a sensitive approach and practical wisdom.[5] The doctor needs to have a 'feel' for the particular situation. Acquiring this 'feel' or perceptual capacity takes time and experience. Rules and guidelines cannot dictate what should happen in every case; the doctor needs to retain a flexibility of approach to adapt to the particular patient's situation. Giving priority to the particular situation lies at the core of practical wisdom. The study of the plays in this book challenges the reader with narratives that involve the deepest emotions.

Aristotle's view of virtue is expressed both in feelings and actions. The virtuous doctor feels appropriately as well as having intellectual competence and is thus able to make a judgement as to what is appropriate to the situation. Intuition and imagination also play a part in practical wisdom. On occasions in situations of uncertainty it can be difficult to explain the reasoning behind some intuitive judgements. The doctor's attention is outwards towards the patient and her compassion a part of her understanding of the patient's particular situation. This understanding of the patient's situation, central to compassion, requires imagination which can be fostered by studies of the arts and humanities.

We will therefore conclude by looking at the question 'What is a good doctor?' in relation to the chapters in *The Silent Treatment*.

COMMUNICATION

Shakespeare shows us in *King Lear* how failure of communication can generate suffering and regret. Cordelia's honesty at the start of the play is misconstrued by the ageing king, who banishes her from his kingdom. This misunderstanding leads to Lear's slow decline into madness and is the catalyst for torture and murder. The king must embark on a journey of self-discovery and rehabilitation, and it is only when the king begins to listen and reflect that he can find a form of resolution and peace.

As in many of the other plays, a strong narrative backbone is provided by the intrafamilial tensions, the unspoken and the assumed. The king is initially unable to see the dynamics at work within his family and is effectively blind to the machinations of Goneril and Regan. Gloucester, too, must endure suffering and physical blinding before he can 'see' the reality of the situation. These problems in communication and understanding provide us with an insight into the consequences of refusing to listen.

The good doctor has a passion for listening and conveys both in this form of silent treatment and when she is talking, that the patient matters. The doctor and patient are above all two human beings. Phillips quotes Winnicott: 'When we are face to face with a man, woman or child in our speciality (psychoanalysis) we are reduced to two human beings of equal status.'[15]

Doctors may be perceived as being in a position of power in relation to the patient, but this superiority is a form of distancing. Superiority can be changed to be viewed instead as a useful difference by adopting a listening position where there is no such thing as superiority, because there is nothing to be superior about.[15] Doctors need to develop an appetite for listening, talking and to be comfortable with disagreement and to enjoy the value of differing perspectives.

Communication involves compassion, which is composed of a number of virtues; the ability to see the world through the patient's eyes (empathy), combined with an urge to do something to help (kindness and generosity) and altruism, which is putting the patient first.

CARE

Harold Pinter's 1960 play *The Caretaker* is a sophisticated exploration of the notion of 'care'. Mick, Davies and Aston all crave 'care' and all three have things to 'care about'. Through the course of the play, Pinter exposes the characters' vulnerabilities, ending with the expulsion of the frail Davies into an 'uncaring' outside world. Yet the play also asks us to consider the 'duty of care'. We learn from Aston that he has been traumatised by a brutal form of shock therapy carried out against his consent, and has since been unable to 'get it together'. Davies, too, is mockingly undermined when Mick offers him the job of 'Caretaker', both demeaning him and raising his expectations.

The play prompts many questions: what do we mean by 'taking care' of

someone? How do we 'take care' of ourselves? Undoubtedly, all three characters suffer in Mick's semi-derelict house. Because the characters are essentially
left without care, they cannot achieve their goals and suffer a form of stasis,
unable to find resolution.

The good doctor is aware of his duty of care, to put the patient first before
any personal interests. Providing care at the end of life is complex and involves
a multidisciplinary team. The doctor should respect the skills of other team
members and be prepared to share the care of the patient. Caring for the patient
involves listening to their psychosocial needs as well as providing competent
diagnosis, investigation and treatment. Medicine is in danger of losing the
vital caring component in the face of pressures from scientific and technological advances which threaten to portray patients as clients or customers with
problems to be solved. Such technical care must always be tempered with
compassion.

Caring for colleagues and caring for oneself are also important qualities of
the good doctor. We have described the syndrome of burnout and discussed
how important it is for doctors to connect with patients and to avoid distancing
themselves from distressing situations. In burnout there is a lack of emotional
engagement with the patient; this is compassion fatigue. In this situation the
doctor reverts to the biomedical model of medicine where the patient is viewed
as a broken machine which needs fixing. The emotional engagement must be
appropriate to the situation; a balance must be achieved to prevent the doctor
becoming too involved and unable to make sound clinical judgements. Setting
boundaries is vital and this can usefully be achieved by doctors who spend time
reflecting on their practice with a mentor. It is difficult to continue to provide
effective end-of-life care without debriefing, reflection and mentoring from a
senior colleague.

CONNECTION

Like Kane's *Blasted*, *Journey's End* depicts a group of individuals attempting
to survive at the limits of human endurance and suffering. Sherriff depicts
the horrors of life in the trenches in great detail, but he is also human in his
representation of the surrogate 'family' of soldiers that have learned coping
strategies to deal with challenges of war. Like any family, there is tension, angst,

arguments and secrets, but ultimately the soldiers form an integrated unit who learn to overcome their differences.

Journey's End also demonstrates the power of silence and the unsaid. Stanhope is desperate to keep his alcoholism a secret from his lover back home. Hibbert complains of neuralgia but is effectively using this to cover his human fear of being killed in the war, and only when Stanhope confesses his own fear is there a sense of resolution as the men decide to 'stick it together'. The flawed Stanhope ultimately displays a deep compassion as he comforts the dying Raleigh at the end of the play. The group learns to cooperate and in this cooperation there is dignity and compassion.

A key theme we have explored is the role of silence, and how silence in both dramatic narrative and medical practice can be more powerful than verbal language, and can have both positive and negative impacts. One factor which may determine whether silence is positive or negative is whether or not it is freely chosen.[12] Further ambiguities around silence complicate the role of listener and speaker. Is the silence in the speaking or the hearing? Silence is more than an absence of sound and can have a dimension which gives the patient space to reflect. It seems that silence is itself a form of communication rather than a lack of communication.[12]

We have looked at the notion of the 'unsaid' – from Joe Keller's unspoken guilt about his negligence to the unspoken love that the two brothers share in *The Caretaker*. As doctors we must learn judgement on when something must be said, and when it is better to remain silent, as silence can sometimes be the best treatment of all.

An essential part of compassion and good communication is the sense of connection with the patient. It only takes a few moments to express interest in another person as a human being, not as a patient. Kindness and attention to giving the patient space and privacy are important if we are to form connected relationships. Silence and eye contact may be powerful tools in establishing connection.

CHOICE

In the chapter on *Antigone*, we examined the notion of choice, and the tensions that exist between autonomy and the expectations of society (these tensions reappear in *Behzti*). Antigone defies the law and gives her 'treacherous' brother a dignified burial, realising that she places herself at the risk of execution by Creon. Yet Sophocles does not simply propose that autonomy is essentially beneficial; instead he demonstrates how choices can set in train a number of different outcomes and that the moral decision by Antigone also causes the death of Antigone's loved ones. We discussed in this chapter the notion of not just a good death but an honourable one. Choice, autonomy and honour are interlinked.

Part of the professional's duty is to seek informed consent from the patient before commencing any treatment. This can involve presenting patients with choices and giving them sufficient time and information so that their medical choices are as informed as any other decisions which they make about their life. Choice implies alternatives, so with choice there may be conflict. Such conflict may be between following what loving relatives are urging them to do, for instance in choosing chemotherapy to 'fight' the cancer rather than pursuing their own preference which might be for a shorter life of better quality. It is part of a doctor's skill to see that merely abandoning the patient and saying 'it's your choice' is not to truly respect their autonomy. Patients need the expert opinion of their doctors, and while they wish to be involved in decision making this may not mean they want to make the decision by themselves but might prefer the doctor to make this choice.

CHANGE

In the chapter on *Little Eyolf*, we examined the notion of change. Medicine is concerned with loss and the dying process is about adapting to change and loss. Sometimes earlier losses such as the loss of status associated with one's occupation may be harder to bear than the dying itself. Patients, families and healthcare professionals often struggle with a prolonged dying process. Change implies uncertainty and this too may be hard to bear. In Western society most people die in hospitals or care homes, not in their home surroundings. Death and dying are unfamiliar to the majority of the public so the doctor can act as a source of help and reassurance to patients and families and enable them to have the important conversations together at the end of life.

For those left behind after the patient's death there is the pain and fear of grief. Doctors can help to normalise the mourning process and also have a responsibility to recognise and treat abnormal grieving.

CONCEALMENT

In the chapter on *All My Sons* we showed how silence and the withholding of information can be damaging, and how the failure to disclose, or to stay silent in the face of untruths can cause the breakdown of the family unit, and by implication a wider society. Joe Keller has lived with the knowledge that his actions have caused the death of a number of soldiers and in effect the death of his own son, Larry. Kate Keller steadfastly refuses to entertain the notion that Larry is dead, as to accept this fact would implicate her husband in his death.

All My Sons demonstrates the human need for transparency, as well as the temptation to remain silent. Joe learns, too late, that he had a responsibility that he neglected in the past, allowing the blame to be shifted to his business partner. But this attempt at 'saving face' has led to a web of lies that has entangled the Kellers' surviving son, Chris. When Joe is forced into a confession, the father feels such shame and dishonour that he takes his own life, thus fragmenting the family and leaving them, perhaps, with more guilt.

The good doctor must have the virtue of honesty. Without the truth the patient becomes more frightened and withdrawn as they cannot make realistic decisions. We have described the subtle ways that collusion can occur between doctors and relatives to hide the truth from patients with the sad result of distancing patients from their families at a time when they need to be close. Collusion can occur between doctor and patient when 'the elephant in the room' is the fact that the patient's impending death is close. Instead of facing this, the patient may undergo futile treatments in a distorted wish to maintain hope. In these situations silence is negative and harmful to the patient.

CRISES

In Sarah Kane's *Blasted* we witness how one's comfortable existence can be shattered without warning. The play intricately maps out how we cope (or fail to cope) with suffering. Ian and Cate are forcibly blown out of their cosseted situation in an expensive hotel and plunged into the horrors of civil war. What they previously took for granted they must fight for with their lives. Ian experiences rape and wounding first hand and must rely on Cate for his survival. The man undergoes a form of transformation from a bullying, swaggering journalist to a vulnerable individual with complex needs.

Blasted teaches us about the potential for compassion in the face of abject suffering. At a moment of crisis, the characters must address their primal needs in order to preserve their dignity. As in *Journey's End*, we see the strength of the human spirit in the face of unimaginable terror and distress, just as Stanhope comforts the dying Raleigh so too does Cate feed the wounded Ian, who in turn thanks her.

Receiving bad news is traumatic and patients react with shock, anger and denial. The professional's role is to be present, allow time to pass and to balance the pace of information giving so that patients can assimilate and adapt to their changed circumstances. We go through life thinking that we are invincible and when faced with impending death we utilise our coping strategies which differ according to our life experiences. Life now is uncertain and precarious so the doctor has a role in providing support, kindness and security. It is a skill to impart the confidence to allow the patient to feel safe in what is clearly an unsafe situation. Providing continuity of care is fundamental to this process; it is another facet of silent treatment.

COMPLEXITY

Caryl Churchill's *Cloud 9* demonstrates how social expectation and prejudice can undermine the individual. We examined how the notion of one's identity can be 'fixed' by others, and expectations of race and gender can be naive and disempowering. Churchill's play investigates paternalism in its many forms, from the hypocritical and overbearing Clive in colonial Africa, to the glib and disingenuous 'acceptance' by Martin of women's rights.

Cloud 9 shows us how we can become a product of our perceived social context and how the way we are viewed can insidiously 'define' our identity and place in society. The play also examines how histories are written, and the temptation to avoid ambiguities as they pose complex questions in favour of making easy categorisations based on old prejudices.

Scientific medicine has combined with market forces to create a new relationship between doctor and patient: that of supplier and customer. Doctors are having to make explicit rationing decisions on individual patients as well as meeting politically defined targets. These reorganisations of health-care have created complicated relationships. Patients make more complaints about their treatments, doctors feel dissatisfied and misunderstood; trust is threatened.

Medicine is a complex discipline and in end-of-life care the complexity is around ethical and psychosocial issues. For instance, on the one hand some members of the public are arguing for euthanasia to be legalised as they believe it will guarantee an easy death while on the other hand doctors are rightly prosecuted if there is any evidence of an attempt to hasten death. There is also widespread criticism of doctors who prolong dying with unnecessary treat-ments, yet when doctors design care pathways to ensure this does not happen they have been accused of shortening the lives of their patients to save hospital beds. Part of the reason for the polarity of these arguments is that since death and dying occur in hospitals and other institutions the public are unfamiliar with the dying process. In this situation it is easy to propagate myths of dread-ful deaths which serve to increase fear and mistrust.

One practical consequence of the complexity of end-of-life care is that doc-tors need to take a pause before making a decision and ensure that they have consulted widely with not only the patient and family but colleagues in the team.

CULTURE

We explored the notion of 'culture' through the play *Behtzi*. In this chapter we examined how a complex framework of loyalties and traditions can be tested by the actions of individuals. *Behtzi* explores how one's faith may be challenged by hypocrisy, secrecy and a debased notion of 'honour'. But the play is humane, and portrays the young Sikh Min with dignity as well as realistically showing the pressure that has been exerted upon her by Balbir, the foul-mouthed mother who has naive faith in Mr Sandhu's 'list'. The tension in the play is generated by the demands of orthodox religion that has been perverted to suit the ends of the senior clerics, resulting in sexual abuse.

The good doctor needs the vision to see the patient in the context of their lives, community and culture. Thus taking account of cultural factors ensures that the patient is first and foremost a person with interests, beliefs, family and friends. In end-of-life care this aspect of care is particularly important since it is only by treating the patient as an individual within their culture that the doctor can understand their wishes for their care. The end of life is a time of reflection as to the meaning of one's existence and a time when questions about what will happen after death are at the forefront of some patients' minds. It is vital that patients are given the opportunity to talk about these subjects if they wish, and to respect their silence if they do not want to discuss these matters. Doctors who let their patients tell their story without interruption elicit more information and patient satisfaction without taking more time.[18]

Doctors have their own medical culture and need to be aware of how this can affect the patient. They may use medical jargon, appear busy and can utilise distancing tactics which can make the patient fearful that they are wasting our time. This attitude may be prevalent in doctors when they become unwell themselves and the good doctor must show generosity and kindness in allowing the sick doctor to be a patient.

COOPERATION

'No man is an island' and nowhere is this truer than in end-of-life care. Care depends on cooperation between the professional family and the patient and their biological family.

The good doctor appreciates the importance of team-working and in particular ensuring that the patient is never dropped from the team. Team-working always involves a potential for conflict, but this should be accepted and indeed welcomed. Doctors should encourage patients and colleagues to express their concerns without necessarily feeling a pressure that they have to solve the problem by themselves.

Patients want competent and humane doctors who will respect them and listen to their views without hurrying them. They want doctors who communicate with kindness and who keep their secrets. They expect a doctor to be honest and open and to treat them as equals. They value a doctor who has the humility to admit uncertainty and vulnerability and who is prepared to share their humanity.[1,8,22]

Medical education helps students to learn new knowledge and skills and to develop professional caring attitudes. It is in this latter task that we believe the medical humanities can play an important role. Encouraging reflective practice requires doctors at every level to re-examine their own values, attitudes and behaviour from the patients' point of view. As Ashcroft comments, 'A code is merely the outward form of medical virtue, not its moral heart. To perceive the moral heart of medicine student and doctors are studying the humanities.'[20]

Holmes suggests that perhaps the key to good doctoring is the ability to see the world through the patient's eyes and to imagine what it must be like to be on the receiving end of our treatment.[21]

Working on Aristotle's theory that if we develop good doctors they will have *phronesis* or practical wisdom, and so make sound ethical decisions, how are medical students and doctors in training to acquire and develop professional virtues? Practical wisdom is not mentioned in medical training; rather, the term clinical judgement is preferred. Practical wisdom is the practised ability to help patients to choose wisely among treatment and diagnostic options.[23] It emphasises the central position of the patient in decision making and acknowledges the ethical dimension to every clinical decision. Practical wisdom incorporates clinical decision making with the patient's views on their goals of care and ethical reasoning. Aristotle suggests that virtue makes us aim at the right target, and practical wisdom makes us use the right means.[24]

Practical wisdom is about aligning the right means with good ends. In virtue ethics practical wisdom (*phronesis*) is directed toward human flourishing (*eudaimonia*). Practical wisdom enables the good doctor to make the right choices by identifying the right means to achieve good ends, through reflection and focusing principles of ethics to specific circumstances. The wise doctor, who has listened to the patient, their family and her colleagues, knows which ends are valuable and how they can be best achieved in a particular context and which virtues and principles of duty are most relevant in a given situation. The good doctor ensures that clinical judgement is not solely the clinician's judgement.[25] Just as doctors are accustomed to reflect when ordering a test, 'How will the results of this test change my management of this patient?', they should add a second question: 'How will this test or treatment help achieve the patient's goal of care?'

The good doctor will ensure that medical interventions only occur when they are appropriate rather than simply because they are available. Doctors function most effectively when they are working in a supportive environment which puts the patient's interests at the centre of care. There is a risk that doctors may become swamped in the bureaucracy of a management culture of targets, formal contracts, mistrust and blame. However, the essence of professional care is the independence of standards of clinical excellence from market values and business contracts.[26] Professionalism can be more positively viewed as a constellation of virtues which patients and society can identify. These will ensure that their doctors will act in their best interests for the appropriate motivation. Through compassionate engagement with the patient the good doctor is able to empathise, listen, interpret and act appropriately in response to the stories and plight of their patients.[27]

REFERENCES

1 Irvine D. The performance of doctors: the new professionalism. *Lancet*. 1999; **353**: 1174–7.
2 Cruess RL, Cruess SR, Johnston SE. Professionalism: an ideal to be sustained. *Lancet*. 2000; **356**: 156–9.
3 Campbell D. Doctors' strike over pensions hits hospitals and GP surgeries. *The Guardian*. 21 June 2012.
4 General Medical Council. *Tomorrow's Doctors*. London: GMC; 2009.
5 Gilles JCM. Getting it right in the consultation: Hippocrates' problem; Aristotle's answer. *Occasional Paper 86*. London: Royal College of General Practitioners; 2005.
6 General Medical Council. *Good Medical Practice*. London: GMC; 2009.
7 Cruess R, Cruess S. Teaching professionalism: general principles. *Med Teach*. 2006; **28**: 205–8.
8 Chandratilake M, McAleer S, Gibson J *et al*. Medical professionalism: what does the public think? *Clinical Medicine*. 2010; **10**: 364–9.
9 Stephenson A, Higgs R, Sugarman J. Teaching professional development in medical schools. *Lancet*. 2001; **357**: 867–70.
10 Rezler AG. Attitude changes during medical school: a review of the literature. *J Med Educ*. 1974; **49**: 1023–30.
11 Elliott D, May W, Schaff PB *et al*. Shaping professionalism in pre-clinical medical students: professionalism and the practice of medicine. *Med Teacher*. 2009; **31**: 295–302.
12 Maitland S. *A Book of Silence*. London: Granta; 2008.
13 Papadakis MA, Teherani A, Banach MA *et al*. Disciplinary action by medical boards and prior behaviour in medical school. *N Engl J Med*. 2005; **353**: 2673–82.

14 Stern DT, Fronha AZ, Gruppen LD. The prediction of professional behaviour. *Med Educ.* 2005; **39**: 75–82.

15 Phillips A. *Equals.* London: Faber & Faber; 2002.

16 Annas J. *Intelligent Virtue.* Oxford: Oxford University Press; 2012.

17 Hursthouse R. Art of life. *Times Literary Supplement.* 21 December 2012. p. 38.

18 Mechanic D. Managing time appropriately in primary care. *BMJ.* 2002; **325**: 690.

19 Paice E, Heard S, Moss F. How important are role models in making good doctors? *BMJ.* 2002; **325**: 707–10.

20 Ashcroft A. Searching for the good doctor. *BMJ.* 2002; **325**: 719.

21 Holmes J. Good doctors, bad doctors: a psychodynamic approach. *BMJ.* 2002; **325**: 722.

22 Coulter A. Patients' views of the good doctor. *BMJ.* 2002; **325**: 668–9.

23 Kaldjian LC. Teaching practical wisdom in medicine through clinical judgement, goals of care and ethical reasoning. *J Med Ethics.* 2010; **36**: 558–62.

24 Aristotle. *Nicomachean Ethics.* Indianapolis: Bobs-Merrill Educational Publishing; 1962.

25 Pellegrino ED. The anatomy of clinical judgements: some notes on right reason and right action. In: Engelhardt HT, Spicker SF, Towers B, editors. *Clinical Judgement: a critical appraisal.* New York: Dordrecht D Reidel Publishing Co.; 1979.

26 Barilan YM. Responsibility as a meta-virtue: truth telling, deliberation and wisdom in medical professionalism. *J Med Ethics.* 2009; **35**: 153–8.

27 Charon R. Narrative medicine: a model for empathy, reflection, profession and trust. *JAMA.* 2001; **286**: 1897–902.

Bibliography

Bhatti GK. *Behzti (Dishonour)*. London: Oberon Books Ltd; 2004.

Churchill C. *Cloud Nine*. In: *Plays 1*. London: Methuen Drama; 1996.

Ibsen H. *Little Eyolf*. William Archer, translator. Stillwell: Digireads.com Publishing; 2008.

Kane S. *Blasted*. Urban K, editor. London: Methuen Drama; 2011.

Miller A. *All My Sons*. London: Penguin Classics; 2009.

Pinter H. *The Caretaker*. London: Faber & Faber; 1991.

Shakespeare W. *King Lear*. Foakes RA, editor. London: Arden Shakespeare; 2007.

Sherriff RC. *Journey's End*. London: Samuel French; 1929.

Sophocles. Antigone. In: *The Three Theban Plays*. London: Penguin Classics; 1984.

Acknowledgements

We would like to thank Gillian Nineham of Radcliffe for her wise advice and patience. We are grateful to the publishing team at Radcliffe for their help in the production of this book, in particular to Camille Lowe and Jamie Etherington.

The chapter on *King Lear* is a reworked version of a paper first published in the *Journal of the Royal College of Physicians of Edinburgh* and we would like to thank Susan Laurence and the editorial team for their consent to publish the work. Thanks, too, to *Medical Humanities* for consent to publish a revised version of the drama workshop. Thanks to Jen Goddard for her help in the Drama workshop and the earlier paper. We would like to thank Therese (Tess) Jones, editor of *Journal of Medical Humanities* for permission to publish work from our paper on Harold Pinter's *The Caretaker*. Thanks too to Rachel Adamson for help with the diagrams.

David would like to thank The Winston Churchill Memorial Trust for their travelling fellowship in 2006, which gave him the opportunity to study attitudes to assisted suicide in the North West of the United States.

We have been inspired by each of the plays we have studied in our book and owe a debt of gratitude to their authors who continue to teach us so much about communicating in a sensitive way.

We thank Pru Jeffrey and Fiona Kerr for their encouragement and support. We acknowledge the many students in Queen's University Belfast and Dundee University Medical School who have taught us so much. The views and errors in this book are our own.

Ewan Jeffrey
David Jeffrey

Index

CPD with Radcliffe

You can now use a selection of our books to achieve CPD (Continuing Professional Development) points through directed reading.

We provide a free online form and downloadable certificate for your appraisal portfolio. Look for the CPD logo and register with us at: www.radcliffehealth.com/cpd

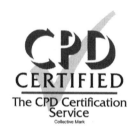